The Official Lamaze® Guide
Giving Birth with Confidence

The Official
Lamaze® Guide
Giving Birth with Confidence

Judith Lothian RN, PhD, LCCE, FACCE
Charlotte DeVries
of Lamaze International

M Meadowbrook Press
Distributed by Simon & Schuster
New York

Library of Congress Cataloging-in-Publication Data

Lothian, Judith.
The official Lamaze guide : giving birth with confidence / by Judith Lothian and Charlotte DeVries.
p. cm.
Includes bibliographical references and index.
ISBN 0-88166-474-X (Meadowbrook Press), ISBN 0-684-03174-4 (Simon & Schuster)
1. Childbirth—Popular works. 2. Natural childbirth—Popular works. 3. Labor (Obstetrics)—Popular works. I. DeVries, Charlotte. II. Title.
RG525.L63 2005
618.4—dc22
                                    2005012963

Editorial Director: Christine Zuchora-Walske
Editors: Angela Wiechmann and Megan McGinnis
Production Manager: Paul Woods
Graphic Design Manager: Tamara Peterson
Cover Photo: © Corbis
Interior Photos: © BananaStock, Ltd; © Brand X Pictures; © Comstock, Inc; © Getty Images;
      © Marilyn Nolt (noltphotos@mail.com).
Index: Beverlee Day

Published by Meadowbrook Press, 5451 Smetana Drive, Minnetonka, MN 55343

www.meadowbrookpress.com

BOOK TRADE DISTRIBUTION by Simon and Schuster, a division of Simon and Schuster, Inc., 1230 Avenue of the Americas, New York, NY 10020

10 09 08 07 06 05   10 9 8 7 6 5 4 3 2 1

Printed in the United States of America

Dedication

To my six granddaughters: Nora, Mary Brigid, Margaret, and Catherine Gibbons, and Margaret and Ellen Lothian. When it is time to birth their babies, I am hoping they will not need to read this book. They will know from their wise, confident mothers about normal birth and will trust, simply and easily, their own power to give birth. —J. L.

To Raymond, Anna, Rocky, and Jesse, who have midwifed me as friend, partner, and mother. —C. D.

ACKNOWLEDGMENTS

Making books, like making babies, takes more than one person. We would like to thank the collective of friends, colleagues, and family members who played important roles in bringing this book to light. Special thanks to Steven Polansky for steerage; to Linda Harmon and the Lamaze International board of directors for their continued hard work on behalf of mothers and babies; to Christine Zuchora-Walske for her patience and keen editing and to the good folks at Meadowbrook Press; to Barbara Bonner and Will Healy for their support in so many ways; to the Institute for Advanced Study in Princeton, New Jersey, where we connected in beautiful surroundings to work on this project; to colleagues and students at the Seton Hall University College of Nursing; to the many women who have written about and modeled normal, natural childbirth with practical knowledge and wisdom; and to Jim and Ray for their loving support and their confidence in our confidence in birth.

PREFACE

WHY ANOTHER BIRTH BOOK?

Well you might ask. There are hundreds of birth books out there already. Some claim to be the "complete guide" or the "better way" to have a baby. Some are filled with illustrations of developing babies, charts listing possible complications, and intricate biological details. Some are technical and scientific; others are warm and even funny.

When we reviewed all these birth books, we noticed that instead of encouraging women, the bestsellers catalog what to fear when you're expecting. It's no surprise that their readers often end up alarmed, afraid, and eager to choose medical interventions like epidurals and cesareans. Very few pregnancy books deliver the simple message that we think pregnant women need to hear most: *Birth is a normal and natural part of life*. We conceived this book from our deep conviction that women know how to give birth—and that women need to rediscover this very important, basic truth.

Throughout history, the wisdom of birthing has belonged to the family and community. The majority of the world's women have given birth among people they know, in a familiar and comfortable place. Birth has been considered a family event, not a medical one—until recently. In our modern, technology-centered culture, birth has moved from the home to the hospital, from the care of friends and family to the oversight of medical professionals, where touch and patience often give way to tests and timekeeping.

We believe deeply that birth is a process you can trust, just as millions of women before you have. This belief isn't sentimental; it's based on our thorough understanding of the physiologic birth process and research that confirms interfering in that process is harmful, unless there's clear evidence that interference provides benefit.

Unlike many other pregnancy and birth books—and, surprisingly, much of standard obstetric care—this book is evidence-based. (For more on evidence-based care, see Appendix A.) We often refer to *The Cochrane Library* (a collection of careful studies and systematic reviews of current research) and *A Guide to Effective Care in Pregnancy and Childbirth* (a summary of *The Cochrane Library*'s maternity research findings with recommendations for practice). As you read this book, you'll see that research supports the excellence of nature's design for birth.

LAMAZE: IT'S NOT ABOUT BREATHING

This book is rooted in the Lamaze philosophy of birth. In the 1950s Fernand Lamaze, a French obstetrician, developed a method of breathing and relaxation that helped women manage childbirth pain. The Lamaze that people have come to know is women puffing and panting their way through labor. But times have changed, and so has Lamaze. What used to be called "the Lamaze method" doesn't really exist today.

Lamaze isn't about breathing techniques anymore. In the years since 1960, when the Lamaze organization began, we've learned many lessons from research and women's experiences of normal, natural birth. As a result, we've changed the content of Lamaze classes. Lamaze is no longer a *method* for giving birth. It's a *philosophy* that educates and instills confidence in women preparing to give birth and become mothers.

In 1960, many women wanted more control of their pregnancy and birth experiences than women typically had at that time. These women wanted their husbands with them during labor and birth; a say in who would attend to their needs; safer, more humane treatment; and more comfortable surroundings for this important life event. Thanks to the efforts of these informed, vocal women who knew things could be better, midwives reemerged as caregivers, labor and birthing rooms became more homelike, and hospitals eliminated some unnecessary routine procedures, like enemas and perineal shaving.

Recently, the birth pendulum has taken an alarming swing backward. Our high-tech healthcare system is designed to look for trouble, and as a result, it labels more and more pregnancies and births as "complicated" or "high-risk." By the end of pregnancy, few women trust their bodies enough to believe they can give birth without drugs and machines. Today we see epidurals used almost routinely, labor induced (started artificially) at epidemic rates, women still confined to their beds in labor and on their backs during birth (the worst position for birthing a baby), and record-breaking numbers of cesarean surgeries performed.

In spite of what women may hear—from their doctors, their hospitals, the media, or the books they read—women *do* know how to give birth simply. And doctors, hospitals, and technology have *not* made birth safer for mothers or babies. We hope this book will help you understand that pregnancy is not a disease requiring medical heroics, and that you, like all women, are well equipped to give birth.

Although the name *Lamaze* will seldom appear in these pages, it's inspired by the plain wisdom of the Lamaze philosophy.

This book is a simple guide for the journey to motherhood. It's written clearly in plain English. It's not an encyclopedia of everything that anyone could possibly know about pregnancy, birth, and breastfeeding. It's not an endless list of obscure and unlikely complications. It's not a textbook laced with clinical terms that ends with a quiz. It's not a guide to medical birth but a guide to normal, natural birth. It encourages you to lay down the heavy burden of what-ifs that can squash confidence. It invites you to replace fear with knowledge, and to build confidence in your ability to give birth on that foundation of knowledge.

In the pages that follow, we'll walk beside you on the path to motherhood. We'll invite you into conversations with other women who've faced the many choices you now face. We'll challenge you to consider which options are right for you and whether standard American obstetric care is conducive

---

The Lamaze Philosophy of Birth

- Birth is normal, natural, and healthy.
- The experience of birth profoundly affects women and their families.
- Women's inner wisdom guides them through birth.
- Women's confidence and ability to give birth is either enhanced or diminished by the care provider and place of birth.
- Women have the right to give birth free from routine medical interventions.
- Birth can safely take place in homes, birth centers, and hospitals.
- Childbirth education empowers women to make informed choices in healthcare, to assume responsibility for their health, and to trust their inner wisdom.

to normal, uncomplicated birth. When you look beyond the menu of options typically offered to expectant mothers, you'll find that birthing a baby is a much more natural event than you may have thought it could be.

We believe that you have the right and the responsibility to get full and accurate information about birth, and to choose what's best for you and your baby based on that information. We believe the facts speak loudly in favor of normal, natural birth, and this book will show you why. It will give you confidence in your ability to give birth and will show you how to achieve as normal and natural a birth as possible.

© Marilyn Nolt

You are not an accident.
Even at the moment of your conception,
out of many possibilities,
only certain cells combined,
survived, grew to be you.
You are unique, created for a purpose.
Go confidently into the days ahead.

CONTENTS

Chapter 1

WHAT IS NORMAL BIRTH?

*We are just one generation away from the days
when a girl grew up on a farm watching the sheep
and pigs give birth. Anyone who saw that year after
year knew that giving birth was a natural process,
a process that could be trusted.*
—Ina May Gaskin

The mission of Lamaze International and this book is to promote,
support, and protect normal birth. We—like midwife Ina
May Gaskin and the millions of other women who have
witnessed and experienced simple, natural birth—believe
that a woman's body is beautifully designed to grow, birth,
and nurture a baby. To work properly, this elegant design
requires patience and trust. A normal birth is one that unfolds
naturally, free of unnecessary interventions. (See Chapter 7.)

NORMAL BIRTH ISN'T THE NORM

Many women are surprised to learn that pregnancy, birth, and breastfeeding happen quite simply for most mothers and babies. But it's true. A woman conceives, and as she moves through her life—often without even thinking about pregnancy—a miracle happens. Cells divide, a tiny heart starts beating, brain and nerves grow. Nature orchestrates a baby's second-to-second development. It also orchestrates the release of hormones that help the mother's body adapt; that trigger labor and birth at just the right time; that help her cope with the pain and work of labor; that prepare her emotionally and physically to feed and care for her baby; and that ensure that her baby is alert and ready to nurse and meet the world.

Women don't need to read books to grow babies. Women shouldn't need to read books or take classes to give birth either. (But these days, a good book or class can be helpful in achieving normal birth. For more on childbirth education, see pages 91–95.) We are designed perfectly for both jobs, with very few exceptions.

Let's be clear. Some labors and births do require intervention. Some women with very long, difficult labors benefit from medication. The few women who don't go into labor by forty-two weeks may need their labors jump-started. Some babies experience distress that mandates immediate intervention. Some pregnant women have preexisting health problems, like diabetes or heart disease, that require treatment affecting labor and birth. But medicalized births should be a very small percentage of all births.

"Someone once told me that having a baby is our way of assisting God in a miracle. I couldn't have said it better myself. My birth experience was important to me because I knew that I had a very specific and important job to do at that moment: to bring my baby into the world as healthy as possible. Every contraction, every breath, every push was bringing me closer to the end result: giving birth to my son. The moment he was born, I realized what a miracle he was, what a miracle conception and birth are to us as parents and to humankind. I felt a kinship with every woman throughout history who has given birth. This is what my body was made to do."

—April

An evolving body of research repeatedly shows the danger of interfering without a valid reason in the natural processes of pregnancy, birth, and breastfeeding. Any intervention, no matter how simple it seems, may disrupt hormone release and create problems that, in turn, must be managed with more interventions. (For more on this "cascade of interventions," see Chapter 4.) In light of such evidence, the World Health Organization (WHO), a leader in the international public health effort to promote normal birth, says that maternity care should aim to achieve a healthy mother and child with the *least* intervention safely possible.[1]

In the United States, reality falls far short of this goal. Most births in the U.S. today are interrupted by procedures designed to start, maintain, and finish labor according to an arbitrary schedule. Few women experience their pregnant bodies unfolding and opening in their own time, in their own way. Ironically, normal birth isn't the norm for American women.

Nearly half of all expectant mothers in the U.S. receive drugs to begin labor, more than half receive drugs to speed up labor, and more than 60 percent receive drugs to dull labor pain. In contrast, pain management strategies that women describe as very helpful, like birth balls and showers and tubs, are rarely available at hospital births.[2] According to the National Center for Health Statistics, more than 90 percent of laboring women have their babies' heart rates tracked continuously by electronic fetal monitors (EFMs),[3] even though no research has shown that routine EFM use keeps babies safer.[4]

> "With my second pregnancy I wanted a normal birth, a process where I would be left alone, to let things take their natural course…. In some profound way, which surprised me, I felt dehumanized by the cesarean I had with my first baby. I felt I had missed out on something, been robbed of something central to being me, in order to make things simpler for somebody else. As I gave birth to my second daughter, despite the pain, I was aware of something eternal in a woman giving birth, surrounded and helped by other women who had given birth themselves. I felt a connection to *life* that I did not feel the first time."
> —Indira

Despite all these "helpful" interventions, the U.S. cesarean rate is at an all-time high: More than 28 percent of American babies are born surgically.[5] This far exceeds the 6-percent rate considered reasonable by the WHO.[6] Although cesarean surgery is safer today than in the past, it still carries significant short-term risks for babies, and both short- and long-term risks for mothers.[7]

We're just beginning to understand the impact of birth practices on breastfeeding, but already it's clear that intervention-intensive labors and routine separation of babies and mothers interfere with nature's plan for babies' easy transition to life outside the womb.[8] Yet despite a wealth of research and history that prove "babies were born to be breastfed"[9] and show the many negative effects on mothers and babies who don't breastfeed,[10] formula feeding continues to be the norm in our society. Women are bombarded with advertising—and other cultural images and messages—that imply formula feeding is just as good as breastfeeding.

PRACTICES THAT PROMOTE NORMAL BIRTH

Research reveals not only the dangers of interfering in the natural process of birth, but also maternity care practices that help keep birth normal. The WHO identifies four care practices, and Lamaze adds two more (marked with asterisks: *).
1. Labor should begin on its own.
2. Laboring women should be free to move throughout labor.*
3. Laboring women should have continuous support from others throughout labor.
4. There should be no routine interventions during labor and birth.*
5. Women should not give birth on their backs.
6. Mothers and babies should not be separated after birth and should have unlimited opportunity for breastfeeding.

We explain each of these care practices in detail and present evidence to support their importance in Chapter 8. These practices ensure the best care for birthing women around the world.

WHY DON'T MORE WOMEN CHOOSE NORMAL BIRTH?

If the facts speak so loudly in favor of normal birth, why don't more women choose it? We believe that because normal birth is uncommon in the U.S., many women either don't know it's an option or don't understand it. If women don't understand the importance of normal birth and breast-feeding, they can't make truly informed choices about the birth and care of their babies.

Here's another way to think about informed choice: Let's say you like the taste of cod and live in a little Midwestern town, where you've grown up content with frozen cod, the only kind your local grocer stocks. But then one summer you take a seaside vacation, and for the first time you taste fresh cod! You discover that the options offered by your grocer back home are very limited. Now you know that eating fresh cod is an entirely different experience from eating frozen cod. When you return home, you persistently ask your grocer for more options in the seafood section, and eventually they become available.

> In spite of the evidence, U.S. maternity care continues to sabotage normal birth rather than support it. In 2002, the *Listening to Mothers* survey learned that among nearly 1,600 new mothers across the U.S., 44 percent had labor induced, 71 percent did not move freely during labor, 93 percent had electronic fetal monitoring, 86 percent had intravenous lines, 74 percent gave birth on their backs, and almost 50 percent of their babies spent the first hours after birth with hospital staff. Only 1 percent of the women experienced all six care practices that promote normal birth, and none of these women gave birth in a hospital.[11]

Our current birth culture is like that little grocery store. Our society sets an array of choices before us, leading us to think, "These are my options. They must be the best available." But there are other options besides what "everyone else" is doing, what your hospital or doctor says is "standard" or "best," and what you've read in magazines or seen on TV.

This book introduces you to those other options. As you read on, you'll learn about the physiology of normal birth and how to keep your birth as normal as possible. You'll also learn how standard U.S. maternity care can sabotage normal birth. This knowledge will give you a strong foundation to make the best possible decisions for you and your baby.

This knowledge will also build your confidence. It'll help you believe that you can trust your body's design as you join the circle of women who have powerfully and simply birthed their babies.

WHY YOU SHOULD BOTHER TO LEARN MORE

Your upcoming birth experience is about much more than getting your baby out of your belly and into your arms. How your birth unfolds will profoundly affect your life, regardless of whether you think it will. It's an event you'll never forget.

Research shows that the day a woman gives birth is not "just another day," and that decades later, women clearly recall positive and negative aspects of their birth experiences.[12] Women's satisfaction with their births has little to do with the length, difficulty, or painfulness of their labors and more to do with their personal expectations, their involvement in decision making, and how they were treated by their caregivers.[13] Even women who are content to let others make decisions (including birth decisions) for them are more satisfied with their births if they're more involved in making birth decisions.[14]

> "I was at a birth recently where the mother was very afraid of needles and pain. As she methodically moved through the stages of birth, she became more and more empowered to believe in her own body and her ability to bring into the world a beautiful, healthy baby boy. Her self-identity will never be the same."
> —Vicki

Your memories of birth can influence your confidence and self-image in the future. Childbirth educator Penny Simkin says, "The potential for positive impact is great, but it takes planning, advance preparation, and safe, respectful nurturing. I'd urge women to take their upcoming childbirth very seriously. It matters too much to turn the experience of a lifetime over to someone else."[15]

Your baby's birth is a life-changing event, and it is *your* experience—not the hospital's, not the doctor's—to remember and cherish. If you seize the opportunity to prepare for and expect a positive birth experience, you'll most likely find that giving birth increases your confidence and strengthens your self-image—which will make you a more capable woman in all aspects of your life. If, instead, you hand over this important event to the direction of others, you'll do nothing to build your self-esteem.

You can make many choices to guide your pregnancy and birth down the path you prefer. You can choose how to care for yourself during pregnancy, where to have your baby, who will help you give birth, how to labor, how to give birth, how to meet your newborn, and how to feed and care for your baby. But even if your pregnancy, labor, and birth don't go as you'd hoped, your positive attitude, your care of your body, and your careful learning, planning, and choosing will build you up.

The first step in learning more about normal birth is looking back at the history of childbirth. A snapshot of the dramatic changes during the last century will help you understand why current U.S. maternity care makes normal birth more difficult for us than it was for our great-grand-mothers. We think it'll inspire you to think about birth in a new way.

Chapter 2

The History
of Birth

Stories have to be told or they die, and when they die,
we can't remember who we are or why we're here.
—Sue Monk Kidd

From Natural to Medical

So much of what we hear and see about birth these days
suggests that women are lacking, that what we bring to birth
isn't enough, that we need technological help to get our
babies born. Listen to a few medical stories about birth,
and you'll probably wonder how women were able to
have babies in past centuries.

But if you investigate the history of birth more closely,
you'll see that once upon a time, birth was a much simpler
process. Ironically, as birth technology has become more
sophisticated, complication and intervention rates have increased.

Medical doctors led childbirth's relocation from the
home to the hospital. Doctors are trained to view the world
as a place where people need curing and fixing, as indeed
many do. But if something isn't broken, it doesn't need to be
fixed. Pregnancy is not a disease, yet many doctors treat it
that way. When obstetricians imposed the "disease model"
on birth, they redefined a very natural, normal event as
risky business.

Until the 1900s, most women gave birth at home with a
midwife's help. In the 1910s and 1920s, medical education
was improving and doctors were becoming more organized
as a profession. As doctors unified, they helped develop laws
that enhanced and protected their own power—especially in
running hospitals. The prestige of medical science grew, and
upper-class women began to seek the care of doctors (who

were usually male). People began to view midwives as backward, suitable only for lower-class women who couldn't afford to have doctors at their births.[1]

The medical establishment fostered prejudice against midwives' intelligence, abilities, training, and skill. Many midwives were immigrants and didn't speak English fluently. Many were poor, many were black, and most were women. They weren't equipped to challenge the campaign being waged against them, and so began a long debate among doctors, government agencies, and midwifery supporters. This argument—which never even started in most of the rest of the world—continues today in the U.S.

So what resulted when birth shifted from homes and midwives to hospitals and doctors? It's hard to compare hospital and home birth statistics fairly, but the death rates of mothers and babies during this period can tell us a few important things.

The period when childbirth shifted from home to hospital did see some positive effects for mothers and babies. The maternal and infant death rates in the United States were high around 1900—as high as today's rates in developing countries. Over the the next forty years, as the overall standard of living improved thanks to better water treatment, housing, and sanitation, the health of mothers and babies followed suit. During that same period, medical advances—specifically, the introduction of antibiotics and blood transfusions—contributed to further dramatic declines in perinatal death rates.[2]

However, medical science had negative effects on mothers and babies during this time, too. To hasten delivery, doctors used procedures and instruments that often harmed mother and baby. Studies show that in the United States, obstetric interference in hospitals was associated with a large increase in baby deaths from birth injuries.[3] Hospitals also harbored germs and allowed practices that led to childbed fever in mothers. A 1925 national study concluded that "untrained midwives approach and trained midwives surpass the record of physicians in normal deliveries."[4]

Even though reports confirmed that midwives were better assistants at normal births, the medical campaign worked. Male doctors became the preferred birth attendants as middle- and lower-class women followed the example of the upper class. Statistics show the grim result: In the 1920s, more mothers and babies died in hospitals than at home births attended by midwives.[5]

Gradually, childbirth came to be seen as an affliction that required medical help, and the womanly art of midwifery gave way to the powerful politics of medicine. By the mid-1930s, most births were happening in hospitals. Despite evidence that told a very different story, doctors convinced women that midwives were dirty, illiterate, and incompetent and declared themselves the only competent baby deliverers. From here on, the home was deemed an unfit place for birth, and birthing women "required" outside help and such "improvements" as twilight sleep (morphine and scopolamine injection), which heavily drugged a laboring woman and erased her memory of birth.

Childbirth's move from home to hospital improved the lives of doctors. In a hospital, one doctor could care for many women at once. Doctors no longer had to travel to mothers' homes and work at inconvenient hours in unfamiliar territory.

This change did not, however, improve the lives of women. It swept away respect for the abilities of both birthing women and midwives. It dried up the flow of empowering birth stories.[6] As a result of twilight sleep, women had no memories of their births to treasure and pass along.

Many people today still view birth as a medical event fraught with danger. "What if something goes wrong?" they ask. "Look how many mothers and babies died in the old days!" they exclaim.

Midwife Ina May Gaskin is quick to differ: "Our bodies *must* work pretty well, or there wouldn't be so many humans on the planet."[7] Of the more than 2,300 babies born at the Farm, Gaskin's midwifery center in Tennessee, 96 percent were delivered without medical assistance.

Indeed, there's no research that shows medical birth is safer for women and babies. Actually, research reveals more risks for mother and baby when the birth team "expects trouble" and where medical intervention is routine.[8]

If you could step into a 1950s American hospital, you'd see women left to labor alone—often drugged and confined to bed—then moved to loud, bright delivery rooms and strapped onto sterile tables, lying on their backs with their feet pressed high overhead in metal stirrups. Gowned and masked doctors and nurses directed these births and typically forbade mothers to have family present and to hold or sometimes even see their babies right after birth. Home birth was becoming a distant memory.

By the 1960s, medicalized birth was so common in the United States that most women didn't know there was any other kind. They routinely labored without support, were given enemas, had their genitals shaved and disinfected, and gave birth on their backs, draped with sterile sheets to prevent them from touching (and possibly infecting) their newborns. Hospital staff whisked the babies away, washed and clothed them, wrapped them in sterile receiving blankets, and put them on display in nurseries far from their mothers. Formula feeding at scheduled times became the norm. Women were told that this was good, modern medical practice.

MOTHERS SPEAK OUT

Luckily, some women didn't accept the medical view of birth, and they spoke out. It began as just a murmur, but as more and more women demanded an active role in birth, their voices grew too strong to ignore. They insisted on—and got—childbirth education and breastfeeding information and support. Their steady work rekindled midwifery and natural childbirth.

In the late 1950s, Marjorie Karmel wrote *Thank You, Dr. Lamaze* after birthing her baby in Paris with Fernand Lamaze at her side. (She'd been inspired to try Lamaze's natural childbirth method after reading Grantly Dick-Read's *Childbirth without Fear.*) When she met Elisabeth Bing in New York City soon afterward, the two women set about teaching as many women as possible to approach childbirth without fear and to learn how to work with their bodies in labor and birth. In 1960, Karmel and Bing established Lamaze International (then called the American Society for Psychoprophylaxis in Obstetrics, or ASPO), one of the most important childbirth organizations in the country.

Like so many other social changes in the U.S., the prepared childbirth movement gained strength as a consumer movement. More and more women and men convinced their doctors and nurses that women would have better births and healthier babies if they were better educated and better prepared for birth. Medication use could be reduced, and women could be awake, in control, and supported by those around them in what could be a more rewarding, less traumatic event for everyone.

More challenges to medicalized birth came in the 1960s. Across the Atlantic, British anthropologist Sheila Kitzinger burst onto the scene with her book *The Experience of Childbirth* in 1962, suggesting that labor pain shouldn't be drugged away, but rather embraced as "pain with a purpose" in the perfect design of birth. American obstetrician Robert Bradley's 1965 book *Husband-Coached Childbirth* stressed the importance of women having their companions present during labor and delivery. In 1967, Elisabeth Bing's *Six Practical Lessons for an Easier Childbirth* became a guide for thousands of women who wanted to prepare actively for birth.

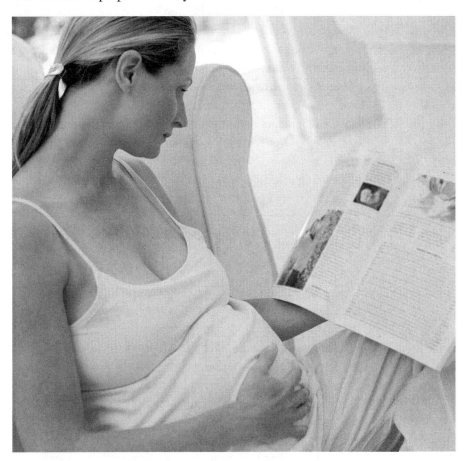

The birth revolution continued in the next decade. The Boston Women's Health Book Collective (a women's health education and advocacy group) published its historic book *Our Bodies, Ourselves* in 1970. This book told women that they had the power to bring about change in women's health and suggested that the medical approach to normal life events like birth might not be effective or healthy. Soon more writers woke up and spoke up with books like Doris Haire's *The Cultural Warping of Childbirth* (1972), Suzanne Arms' *Immaculate Deception* (1975), and Ina May Gaskin's *Spiritual Midwifery* (1975).

As like-minded women around the country sought out one another and made birth choices not offered in hospitals at the time, they angered the medical community by challenging its long-standing authority. Elisabeth Bing recalls, "The fight for recognition of the idea of family-centered maternity care, in which fathers and children become part of the birth experience, was a slow and hard fight. Acceptance did not come overnight. I remember well how I was told that surely this was all a fad, that women would soon forget, and that ideas as strange as encouraging a woman to be awake and aware while giving birth were beyond all rational thinking."[9]

Governments and healthcare systems were indeed slow to react. But the evidence supporting a move toward more natural birth was so strong that even bureaucrats and members of the very profession being criticized were compelled to respond. In 1975, Uruguayan obstetrician Roberto Caldeyro-Barcia, who later served as president of the International Federation of Gynecology and Obstetrics, advocated getting laboring women off their backs and out of stirrups and allowing women to labor in their own chosen positions.[10] In the late 1970s, U.S. congressional hearings called for reducing the alarmingly high cesarean rate and for improving prenatal care around the country. During the same decade, French obstetrician Michel Odent's research led him to promote the use of showers and baths for comfort during natural birth.[11] In the late 1980s, the Carnegie Foundation for the Advancement of Teaching made midwife recruitment and education recommendations that highlighted the importance of and growing demand for midwife care.[12] In 1992, the United Kingdom's

House of Commons finally admitted that research showed the home to be as safe as a hospital for birth and that, in fact, home birth *should* be a publicly supported option.[13]

Meanwhile, across the North Sea, women in the Netherlands have enjoyed watching the international birth pendulum swing back and forth. The Dutch government has supported midwife-assisted home birth for decades. A third of Dutch births happen at home, and nearly half of Dutch women have their babies with midwives in attendance. The Netherlands consistently ranks among the top countries in the world for successful birth outcomes, along with Japan, Iceland, Sweden and Finland.[14]

OBSTETRICS UNDER THE MICROSCOPE

The Cochrane Group Is Born

In 1979 Archie Cochrane, then director of a prestigious epidemiology research unit in the UK, identified obstetrics as the medical specialty with the worst record for using randomized, controlled trials (the gold standard in research) to evaluate the effectiveness of patient care. Three obstetrician-epidemiologists took on the challenge of changing that: Murray Enkin from Canada, Iain Chalmers from the UK, and Marc Keirse from the Netherlands.

The efforts of Enkin, Chalmers, and Keirse produced *The Cochrane Library*[15] (a collection of careful studies and systematic reviews of current research) and *A Guide to Effective Care in Pregnancy and Childbirth*[16] (a summary of *The Cochrane Library*'s maternity research findings with recommendations for practice). Currently more than nine thousand controlled trials from almost four hundred medical journals, in eighteen languages from eighty-five countries, are registered in *The Cochrane Library*, which is available electronically and is constantly updated. Its research team includes doctors, midwives, nurses, public health experts, and statisticians who find and evaluate the world's best research and then make recommendations for practice.

A Guide to Effective Care in Pregnancy and Childbirth (see Appendix A) classifies maternity care practices as:
- beneficial
- probably beneficial
- both risky and potentially beneficial
- of unknown effectiveness
- probably not beneficial
- probably ineffective or harmful

Thanks to *The Cochrane Library*, caregivers now have easy access to high-quality research and can provide evidence-based care to women and their babies. Nonetheless, most U.S. obstetricians still don't consistently base their practices on best evidence.

The Role of Technology

Why, when research continually supports normal, natural birth and shows the danger of routine birth interventions, does birth remain stuck in the realm of medicine? We think it's trapped there by the same force that has made computers, cell phones, and GPS so popular. There's no doubt that technology *can* improve our lives, but it doesn't *always* do so. Any device, drug, or procedure can cause either good or bad results. Using technology just because we can often leads to unintended consequences.

Modern medical technology routinely changes how birth is meant to proceed. Here are just some of the routine interventions that often divert mothers from normal, natural birth:
- **Prenatal tests** are often misinterpreted, causing unnecessary stress, loss of confidence, and sometimes misinformed decisions.
- **Drugs** can begin a woman's labor on the spot, even though her body and her baby may not be ready for birth. They can also intensify labor, which may necessitate other drugs to help manage her pain if contractions get too intense.
- An **epidural** removes a mother's labor pain, but also scrambles her body's signals and disrupts the natural course of labor. The medication used in epidurals also affects her baby.

- **Electronic fetal monitoring (EFM)** records a baby's response to labor. External EFM, the most common type, is held against a mother's abdomen with a belt. The belt is connected to a large machine that limits the mother's ability to move around. Research shows that medical staff interpret EFM information inconsistently. (Some research shows that the confinement required for EFM actually *causes* the problems EFM records.) If the information is misread, staff may intervene further, disrupting the normal flow of labor and birth even more.

> EFM certainly *seems* like a good idea. A machine that measures and records a baby's response to contractions provides scientific data about a particular woman's labor. Logic says—and many people assume—that EFM improves birth outcomes.
>
> Actually, three decades of research shows that EFM *doesn't* improve birth outcomes. When EFM is used during labor, no fewer babies die and no fewer have problems at birth. However, more women have cesareans when EFM is used.[17] If EFM doesn't help babies and puts mothers at higher risk of surgical intervention, it is *not* safer care.
>
> In 1988, a Harvard Medical School report described EFM as a "failed technology" but also predicted that doctors wouldn't stop using it because they fear being sued.[18] Fear of malpractice litigation is pervasive in obstetrics. Doctors too often make patient care decisions based on their fear of a lawsuit rather than on evidence-based standards of practice established by their profession.

- A **scheduled cesarean** is faster and more convenient for a doctor and mother than allowing the mother to labor when and for as long as her body might need to. But a cesarean is surgery, and like all surgery, it carries risks for mother and baby that most women don't realize. (See page 154 and 269.)
- **Newborn care procedures and equipment**, such as tests, shots, and warmers (isolettes), often separate mothers and babies. But we know that a mother's warm arms provide the perfect setting for her newborn baby's first hours.

Albert Einstein looked at the state of the world late in his career and said, "It has become appallingly obvious that our technology has exceeded our humanity." We think Einstein is right. As we increasingly pursue and rely on birth technology—that force we've come to trust as faster, safer, better—we not only forget what normal birth is, we also forget how to respond to birth with humanity and patience.

Much of modern birth technology has not improved birth outcomes in the United States. Forty-one countries have lower infant mortality rates than the U.S.[19] The countries with the lowest infant and maternal death rates share, among other practices, a reliance on midwives for primary care at most births.[20] Research suggests that doctors may not be the best birth attendants,[21] and history shows that until the early 1900s they never attended complication-free births.

Obstetricians are trained to diagnose and treat disease and complications in pregnancy and childbirth. They do this extremely well. Medical advances like the development of antibiotics, the diagnosis and treatment of pregnancy-induced hypertension, and the use of blood transfusions have done a lot to reduce maternal death and disease rates.

But doctors are not trained to understand and trust the natural process of birth. They're trained to expect trouble and to manage birth rather than let it move at its own pace. An obstetrician's expertise at fixing problems may make him or her less cautious about disrupting the natural process than a midwife would be. Many obstetricians fear litigation more than intervention. American lawyers and jurors tend to equate good medicine with interventions and technology rather than evidence-based standards of practice. Obstetricians are stuck between a rock and a hard place.

As a result, we perpetuate a system of intervention-intensive birth that too often puts mothers and babies at risk. Childbirth educator and author Penny Simkin warns, "I think we're fiddling with a process that is showing us more and more that it really shouldn't be fiddled with, except where there is clear indication that something is wrong."[22]

SUPPORT FOR NORMAL BIRTH TODAY

Midwives

According to both the American College of Nurse-Midwives (ACNM) and the Midwives Alliance of North America (MANA), a midwife recognizes pregnancy and birth as normal processes and believes the education and empowerment of pregnant women are just as important as good prenatal care.[23]

Midwifery training focuses on understanding and protecting what is normal and natural in pregnancy and birth, while obstetric training focuses on understanding and looking for complications. Holding a midwifery textbook in one hand and an obstetrics textbook in the other illustrates the different outlooks of the two professions: The obstetrics text is much heavier, since it's full of descriptions of rare complications.

One midwife says, "There's a lot of pressure on midwives, particularly if you're hospital-based, to become like hospital residents, to see as many patients as possible and keep pushing people through." But that's not what midwife care is about. Doctor visits average eight or nine minutes per patient.[24] A midwife will tell you that her routine prenatal visit takes up to thirty minutes. The medical part of this visit—checking blood pressure, listening to the baby's heartbeat, and measuring the mother's belly—takes only about four minutes. The rest of the time is for building relationship, trust, and confidence—for getting to know a woman, answering questions, alleviating fears.

Unfortunately, time isn't the only aspect of midwifery that's being threatened by developments in medicine. The very future of midwifery is at risk. Midwifery centers across the country are being forced to close because their malpractice insurance is getting too costly (though midwives are rarely sued) and because obstetricians are refusing to offer backup support to midwives (a legal requirement in most states)—partly because of *their* huge malpractice costs.

Just as parents needed to organize into a consumer movement to improve childbirth in past decades, midwives have realized the need to speak and work together to change harmful legislation and discriminatory practices. As more women choose midwives as caregivers and share their empowering birth stories, the demand for midwives continues to grow in the United States. Midwifery programs around the country continue to train new midwives each year, despite the political pressures working against them.

Other Birth Advocacy Groups

The list of North American organizations advocating for normal birth is ever-growing. In 1994, Lamaze International hosted a gathering of individuals representing more than fifty of these organizations to discuss how to improve care for birthing women and their babies. This meeting gave birth to the Coalition for Improving Maternity Services (CIMS), a group that works to improve birth outcomes while reducing the cost of maternity care.[25] CIMS has developed a Mother-Friendly Childbirth Initiative (MCFI) that hospitals, birth centers, and home birth services can implement to offer the best possible care for both mothers and babies.

The MCFI is based on the following principles. (For the full text of the MCFI, see Appendix B.)

- Birth is a normal, natural, and healthy process.
- Women are empowered when they receive sensitive, respectful care.
- When women are accurately informed of their options in birth, they will make good choices.
- Routine tests, procedures, drugs, and restrictions on laboring and birthing women should be avoided.
- The interests of mothers and babies should come first in maternity care.
- Any maternity care practice should be backed by evidence that it is best for mother and baby.

CIMS works to educate pregnant women as well as professionals and offers a "mother-friendly" designation to hospitals, birth centers, and home birth services that implement the MCFI. Unsurprisingly, CIMS supports the work of midwives because of their long history of promoting, protecting, and supporting normal birth.

Working alongside CIMS in supporting and promoting normal birth are dozens of more specialized groups of nurses, midwives, childbirth educators, and doulas (professionals who support birthing women and their families). Here are just a few:

- The **Association of Nurse Advocates for Childbirth Solutions (ANACS)** helps nurses initiate evidence-based nursing practices that promote normal birth and improve maternity care. ANACS envisions a future "when all childbirth professionals will support women in their childbirth choices, and nurses will all practice evidence-based maternity nursing" with as few interventions as possible.[26]

- **DONA International** (formerly Doulas of North America) believes in the highest quality of emotional, physical, and educational support for women and their families during and after childbirth. DONA has trained about three thousand doulas in evidence-based programs that teach the importance of continuous support for child-bearing women. Doula Christina McGhee explains the value of her work: "I strongly believe that the support of another woman through pregnancy, labor, and postpartum has a profound impact on the health and happiness of the mother, the baby, and the family unit."[27]

- The **Maternity Center Association (MCA)** has been dedicated to improving maternity care since 1918. Among many other firsts, MCA opened the first U.S. school of nurse-midwifery in 1931 and established the first free-standing American birth center in 1975. It continues to be a strong voice in birth research and advocacy. Maternity Wise, MCA's newest major program, promotes evidence-based maternity care. On its website (http://www.maternity wise.org) MCA offers free downloads of many documents that help mothers make informed decisions, such as the Cochrane Collaboration's *A Guide to Effective Care in Pregnancy and Childbirth* (see Appendix A) and the MCA's own *Listening to Mothers* survey, *The Rights of Childbearing Women* (see Appendix C), and *What Every Pregnant Woman Needs to Know about Cesarean Section 2004.*

- Lamaze International launched the **Lamaze Institute for Normal Birth** in 2003 to support initiatives that provide credible, relevant, and useful information about normal birth.[28] The vision of the Institute is that women who are truly informed, confident, and supported will want normal birth and that caregivers should respect the birth process and not intervene without compelling medical reasons. The Institute has developed six evidence-based practice papers. Adapted from the work of the World Health Organization (WHO), these papers provide evidence in favor of care practices that promote, protect, and support normal birth. (See Appendix D.)

THE HISTORY OF BIRTH IS FULL OF STORIES

We Are Family

In the first part of this chapter, we give a brief overview of the history of birth in the U.S. Many historians and anthropologists have also chronicled the global story of birth throughout the ages. Despite the cultural flourishes associated with time and place, it's remarkable how universal the experience of pregnancy and birth is—how much a pregnant North American woman shares with a pregnant Asian woman today, how physically and spiritually similar pregnancy was for a Kenyan woman in the late 1900s and a Victorian Englishwoman. No matter where or when it happens, pregnancy brings with it special clothing and foods,

changes in relationships, growth in maturity and inner strength, and a gathering of helpers who share their wisdom and profoundly touch both mother's and baby's lives.

In the South Pacific island nation of Fiji, a whole community takes responsibility for the pregnancy of one of its women; everybody participates somehow in household preparation, labor, delivery, and postpartum care, providing support and encouragement to the growing family. In the Netherlands, a family and midwife get to know each other as they prepare the home for birth together. In Mexico, a midwife does simple exercises with an expectant mother to encourage her and help her get ready for labor. In New York, a pregnant woman gathers a simple wardrobe for her newborn, laundering and folding tiny socks and sleepers as she longs for the day she'll meet her little one face to face.

Sharing Birth Stories

All birthing women are part of the same circle of mothers. When we share our stories, our wisdom, and our encouragement, we offer each other important tools for navigating our lives. In the realm of birth, we can learn from each other the purpose of labor pain, the rewards of those brief and intense hours that lead to cradling a baby. We can help each other give birth with confidence, thereby gaining strength for future challenges along life's journey. New birth stories are created every hour around the world—stories about unique women in unique situations bringing unique human beings into the world. Every story is special; every one is important.

In 1988, Kathryn Hall founded Birthing Project USA (BPUSA) in Sacramento, California,[29] to help at-risk African American pregnant women invest in their pregnancies and understand the importance of the hard work they're doing in pregnancy. Today, BPUSA pairs pregnant women across the U.S. with volunteer "sister friends" to improve the health and well-being of the young mother and her baby. BPUSA is a modern model of women helping women successfully enter the dance of motherhood.

Children grow up treasuring the stories their parents have repeated to them. Knowledge of our past helps us understand who we are and where we've come from. In the same way, the sharing of birth stories reminds women of their shared strengths, hopes, and fears.

Even if you'll never hear a birth story from your mother or grandmother, there are numberless sources you can—and should—tap. You need birth information told from a variety of perspectives, and what you read in a memoir or hear from a trusted sister, aunt, or friend may be dramatically different from what you read in a birth manual, see in the media, or hear from a doctor.

"It was autumn 1912 when my mother was born to a German housewife, the ninth baby to enter the world in the cramped bedroom of her little Ohio farmhouse. There was no doctor present, no hospital in the sparsely settled area, no running water or electricity on the farm, no time for my grandmother to delight in her newborn. All too soon the care of her family, home, orchards, and garden pulled her back onto her feet.

In the same little town in 1949, my mother birthed me, her third and final child, in a scopolamine haze at the 'modern' hospital two blocks from her little house. A black-and-white hospital photo shows me swaddled in receiving blankets and sleeping in a little nursery box, a hand-printed sign reading 'Baby Jones' above my head. My mother could recall nothing about the night I was born. It was two weeks before she could leave her room to gather me in her arms and take me home.

In 1980, my mother stood in the living room of my little California house. It was the middle of the night, and she was cradling the baby boy I had just birthed with the quiet help of my midwife, my husband, and a trusted friend. Our son had already nursed, moments after he'd come into our world. The dimly lit room was shimmering with the holiness of his arrival.

Three generations of women—my grandmother, my mother, and me—did what women from the beginning of time have done. We stepped into the dance of motherhood in a changing world. We brought our histories, our gifts, and all our strength to those moments when new human beings emerged from our bodies and breathed air into their tiny lungs."

—Charlotte

Here are some questions you might want to ask other women who've given birth:

- How did you feel when you found out you were pregnant?
- Who did you tell first?
- What do you remember about your pregnancy?
- Were you able to talk about your pregnancy with others?
- Did you feel supported or alone during those months?
- Who was your caregiver?
- How did you choose your caregiver?
- How did you prepare for birth?
- Where did you have your baby?
- Who was in the room with you, and what did they do?
- How did your labor start?
- How did you feel and what did you think about during labor?
- What was done to you during labor and birth?
- What were your thoughts when you first saw your baby's face?
- What was it like to breastfeed for the first time?
- If you didn't breastfeed, why not?
- Was becoming a mother what you thought it would be?

Like most conversations, your sharing of thoughts and questions about birth will lead you down interesting pathways to new destinations. You may learn more than you were looking for. Perhaps you'll learn not only about pregnancy, labor, and birth, but also about caring for newborns, about mothers' feelings during those first days postpartum, about the presence or absence of fathers, or about how birth affects relationships. The possibilities are limitless.

Starting Your Own Story

The story of pregnancy and childbirth plays on in your body, as it does in all the women around the world who are pregnant alongside you now. Each story is worth telling, worth hearing, worth treasuring. Your story is no exception. It deserves a place of honor right next to all the stories of parents who, as children's advocate Fred Rogers said, "have loved us into being."[30]

No matter how well you understand the physical process of birth, it still holds a spiritual spark. How you decide to picture your pregnancy is an important choice. Is it a mechanical event that needs modern medicine to help it along? Or is it a natural unfolding of life and of your family history? Your answer to this question is sure to influence the course of your story.

Today, the stories of many births languish in medical files, written in scientific terms that too often increase fear rather than self-confidence. When birth stories are encoded in medical language, the truth about natural birth and the strength of women is usually lost.

You can prevent your story from being lost by sharing it with friends, family, and your child. You can ask those present at your baby's birth to write down what they've witnessed and give their tales to you for safekeeping. You can tell and read the stories on your child's birthday each year, affirming your child's worth and the importance of his or her entry into history. Such birth stories become treasures to children and parents alike. Remember that your birth story isn't just *your* story. It's also your *baby's* story. It's a story of new beginnings for you, for your family, and for the new person who's come into the world through you.

AND NOW THE CHOICES

This slow and powerful work of pregnancy, birth, and helping your child grow up is a beautiful and important bit of weaving in the fabric of humanity. It's a holy event that will be remembered, shared, and used in ways you can't predict, in a world you can't always understand. As U.S. Supreme Court Justice Sandra Day O'Connor says, "We don't accomplish anything in this world alone...and whatever happens is the result of the whole tapestry of one's life and all the weavings of individual threads from one to another that creates something."

The threads of your own life began thousands of years ago when your ancestors brought their offspring safely into this world. Generation followed generation, and here you are today, ready to take your place in the tapestry of life and send another thread into the future through your child.

It's time to make a choice. Because of the way maternity care has evolved in this country, you have two distinct options regarding how to view your pregnancy and birth. What you choose to believe about your ability to grow, birth, and nurture your baby will determine the color and pattern of your piece of the tapestry.

Chapter 3

EARLY PREGNANCY

Rely on your own inner resources,
trust your body's responses, and take joy
in preparing for the new life that is now
becoming a part of yours.
—Peggy O'Mara

The growth of your baby inside you is a natural and self-sufficient process. Perhaps the best thing you can do for both of you is pay attention. Listen to what your body tells you about how to care for yourself, how to prepare for your baby's arrival, and how to give birth. You don't need to be a genius or highly educated to hear and follow your inner wisdom. It's a simple matter of letting nature's perfect design unfold.

Sometime during your pregnancy you'll probably hear or read the word *gestate*, which means "to carry in the uterus from conception to birth." *Gestate* also means "to conceive and develop in the mind." Your pregnancy is the gestation not only of a baby, but also of ideas, attitude, and self-image. It's an opportunity to learn more about your strengths and abilities. At the moment you discover you're pregnant, you embark on this journey of physical and mental growth.

MESSAGE FROM YOUR BODY: "YOU'RE PREGNANT"

What was your first clue? Perhaps you missed a period, or you just had a hunch, or your belly felt sort of "busy." Maybe you sensed something different about your body, little changes you'd never noticed before. Or you found your emotions were strung a little tighter than usual. You wondered: "Could I be pregnant?"

Whether you confirmed your pregnancy with a home test or at a clinic, you likely knew beforehand that *something* was different by observing your body closely. That's just the first of many opportunities pregnancy offers you to be mindful—to pay close attention to your body, your environment, and your instincts. Being mindful during pregnancy is important because it helps you navigate the moments of your day.

During early pregnancy every moment is packed with drama. Beginning at conception (when egg and sperm join), your body undergoes an avalanche of change in a very short time. Even before the embryo (what your baby is called through eight weeks gestation) implants in your uterus, HCG (human chorionic gonadotropin, the hormone detected by pregnancy tests) levels rise. This is the beginning of hormonal changes that continue throughout pregnancy and breastfeeding. These hormonal shifts and your growing baby change your body in amazing ways.

If you take a quiet moment to stand before the mirror after a bath, you might note some changes in your breasts—darker, bigger, bumpier nipples; blood vessels you don't remember seeing before; a feeling of tenderness or heaviness. These early developments in your breasts are your body's first preparations for milk production.

You may be experiencing nausea in the mornings, at mealtimes, or more often. Pregnancy nausea (often called morning sickness) varies from woman to woman, and it can be unpleasant. Eat and drink whatever you think might help you deal with nausea—small, regular snacks that sound comforting and digestible. Take note of what goes down easily. For many women it's carbohydrates.

Research shows that about two-thirds of all pregnant women have some nausea, and that it may actually serve an important purpose: protecting mother and baby from harmful chemicals and food-borne illness.[1] Certain foods are common triggers for pregnancy nausea; many expectant mothers feel sick when they consume or smell eggs, poultry, fish, meat, alcohol, or caffeinated beverages. A pregnant woman's body might perceive these items as threats to an embryo that hasn't finished making a good, strong attachment. (In the same way, her body might crave certain foods because it needs those nutrients.)

If you're suffering from pregnancy nausea, one way to cope is to think of your baby getting strongly established in you, making his or her presence known, helping your body adjust to his or her needs. You might also keep this in mind: One researcher has said that the term *morning sickness* should really be changed to *wellness insurance*; pregnancy nausea may be linked to better birth weights for babies. If nothing else works, keep your eyes on the road ahead: Morning sickness *will* end eventually. For most women, it goes away somewhere between the third and fourth month.

The first weeks of pregnancy are a time of deep tiredness for lots of women. Jennifer remembers wanting to crawl under her desk for a ten-o'clock nap at work: "Those mornings, I'd long to curl up and sleep—just out of the blue. It suddenly occurred to me that I'd *never* been like that! I'm a dancer, full of energy, ready to take on the day. That was my first real attention grabber." Since Jennifer's periods had never been regular, her tiredness was her first signal to begin looking for other changes in her body.

Some women's emotions send them strong signals. You might find yourself snapping back in reply to a casual comment or ready to cry over some small matter. This sensitivity is a message from your baby: "Listen up! We've got work to do together, and I need your attention."

When you pay attention to your body's signals, you'll find them to be valuable information suppliers and bond builders. Midwife Pam England says that while a baby grows inside you without much effort from you, "the development of your parent-identity is not necessarily an automatic process of nature. If you want to help this happen, you'll have to play an active part."[2] As you listen and respond to your unborn baby's messages, you begin a lifetime of conversation with and learning from each other.

WHAT'S HAPPENING?

You and Baby Are in This Together

Pregnancy is not just the making of a baby. It's also the making of a mother. A mother's body and soul grow and adjust to parent each unique child she carries. During pregnancy mother's and child's bodies, rhythms, abilities, and cues develop together. For example:

- Your baby's heart, which begins beating three or four weeks after conception, is growing into the heart of the child you'll raise. Meanwhile, *your* heart is growing into the heart of the mother who'll love this unique human being.
- Your baby's eyes, which are protected by eyelids eight weeks after conception, are becoming eyes that'll behold the world as no other eyes have. Meanwhile, *your* eyes are becoming those of a mother who will see what no one else sees in this new person.
- Your baby's ears, which can hear your voice perhaps as early as nineteen weeks after conception,[3] will enter the world listening for familiar sounds. Meanwhile, *your* ears are developing into those of a mother attuned to the unique voice of this child.

You may hear the word *trimester* (period of three months) a lot while you're pregnant. The division of pregnancy into three chunks of time provides a framework for thinking about your baby's growth and changes in your body.

During your first trimester, what started out as a microscopic ball of cells is rapidly developing into a complete body with facial features and teeth and fingerprints, a full collection of systems from digestive to nervous, and the ability to move and feel. Your baby is nourished through his or her umbilical cord, which is attached to an organ called the placenta, which develops after the fertilized egg implants in the wall of your uterus.

In the first three months of pregnancy your uterus grows to accommodate your growing baby. At about ten weeks you can feel the top of your uterus in your lower abdomen. (By the end of pregnancy, your uterus will be just under your ribs!) Your growing uterus and your high progesterone (pregnancy hormone) levels over the next months will cause a wide variety of physical changes. Even before you gain any weight, you'll notice your waist thickening as your ligaments loosen to help your belly expand. You may urinate more frequently. Your skin may look radiant, or you may develop acne. You may notice that your hair has never looked better. You may find that your breasts are larger, your nipples more erect, and your areolas darker. Your body is already preparing for breastfeeding.

About Due Dates

Calendars can be so comforting—helping us move through the paces of daily life and plan ahead for important events. Circling your baby's due date on your calendar can help you organize your preparations, can make your future more real and exciting, and can help your caregiver manage his or her schedule. But predicting *exactly* when your baby will arrive is not possible.

Though you and your caregiver might calculate a due date forty weeks from the first day of your last period, bear in mind that only about 5 percent of babies arrive on their due dates. Many factors make due dates difficult to pin down. For example, the formula described above assumes a woman has a twenty-eight–day cycle and ovulates on day fourteen, which isn't true for many women. And some babies just take more or less than forty weeks to be ready for the outside world.

Imagine making of a batch of popcorn. Most of the kernels pop during a few noisy moments. But there are lots of early and late poppers, too. All the popped kernels are perfect—but each needs a slightly different amount of time to be fully cooked. The same is true for babies.

Some caregivers are in a hurry to begin labor when they think a baby is fully developed. But only your baby knows when he or she is ready to be born. Your baby's chemistry communicates with yours to declare that all systems are go and that labor should begin. By adopting a relaxed attitude about your due date in early pregnancy, you're practicing patience and trust that'll serve you well as your pregnancy progresses.

WHAT CAN YOU DO?

The beauty of pregnancy is that for most women it just happens. As you go about your everyday life, a miracle occurs within you. Even if you know little about pregnancy and haven't seen a doctor or midwife, your body changes and your baby develops. You're creating a baby all by yourself.

Though pregnancy may not affect your daily routine much, you may view everyday events through a different lens. You may find your good and bad moods more pronounced. Your sleep patterns and dreams may change. Your appetite and your likes and dislikes may shift. Lovemaking may take on different meaning.

You may be wondering, "If pregnancy 'just happens,' is there anything I can *do* to support it?" Yes. You can use the brief days of gestation to discover your strengths, to live well, and to change habits that might be damaging. The most important thing you can do to ensure a healthy you and a healthy baby is to stay healthy yourself. Eat well, rest, exercise, manage stress, and make time for fun.

Handle the Worry Habit

An old Swedish proverb says, "Worry gives a small thing a big shadow." Perhaps it's pregnancy's boost of emotional energy that feeds the specter of worry. No matter how fit you may feel, how much you may enjoy being pregnant, or how radiant you may look, worry can find a way to sneak into your psyche.

Worry is an equal-opportunity ghost; it'll haunt any thought, any insecurity, any issue at all. You may worry about being up to the task of parenting. You may worry about how profoundly becoming a parent will change your life. You may worry about how you look and if you'll ever feel like you again. You may worry about how your child is developing, how you'll handle the pain and hard work of labor, how you'd cope with the hundreds of scary scenarios that come to your attention via conversation and the media.

You know that bristling feeling you get when someone says offhandedly, "Oh, c'mon, don't worry!" Not worrying is easier said than done, especially about matters of pregnancy and birth. After all, worry is a normal emotion and does serve a useful purpose. Naming your fears and examining them can help you understand them, put them in perspective, and develop coping strategies. If your nightmares come true, how might you respond? How might your partner or caregiver help you? How might you prevent or accept or improve the situation?

By all means, face your fears—but don't exaggerate them. Humans tend to grow their worries—to become preoccupied with possible pitfalls, rather than positive probabilities. We've all come through times of great worry in our lives, when fear overtook our thoughts and robbed us of peace and joy. Looking back on those times, we can see that our worries didn't change the eventual outcomes, and that we survived the challenges that felt insurmountable at the time.

Check In with Yourself Daily

Finding the time, energy, and peace to face your fears—or do anything that requires mental focus—is a challenge in our culture. One pregnant woman shared that after years of working at her office, she'd tuned out the sounds of phones ringing and computers clicking. She didn't even notice how noisy her office was until an older coworker looked at her across the bank of desks and said, "You're bringing this child into a world of sounds my babies never heard."

It's true: In just a decade or two, technology has changed the world dramatically. From cell phones to ATMs, from microwave ovens to online grocery stores, from DVDs to TiVo, technology fills our days with vivid images and messages. It's a noisy, busy world that can crowd out the peace we need to connect with ourselves.

Connecting with yourself is an important task during your pregnancy. It's a big job to pay attention to all the physical, emotional, and spiritual changes you're experiencing. It takes concentration to envision a future that includes a new role and a new person. Finding a place of stillness for a few moments each day can help you do this crucial work.

Even if your space and your schedule are crowded, you can find a place and time to keep a daily appointment with yourself. Perhaps you can retreat to the corner of your bedroom, the bathroom, a closet, or an empty room at your workplace.

Perhaps you can sneak a moment before others wake up, after they've gone to bed, before you get in the shower, or during your lunch break. You might want to "check in" at the same time each day so you treat this appointment with yourself as the important time it is.

Your daily check-in may be a few moments of silence, meditation, or prayer. You can use this time to get in touch with not only your feelings, but also your body and the little one who is taking up more and more of it. Close your eyes for a moment and listen to your breathing, then take an inventory of yourself: Are there any tense areas in your body—neck, shoulders, throat, hands, back? Is anything nagging at your mind? Doing a full-body and -mind check will help you identify what needs to be released, relaxed, or dealt with.

Exercising is an excellent way to keep your mind and body healthy during pregnancy. It aids digestion, improves your mood, keeps you fit for the work ahead, and helps you sleep better. Must you exercise to have a healthy baby? No. Are you likely to feel better if you stay active? Yes.

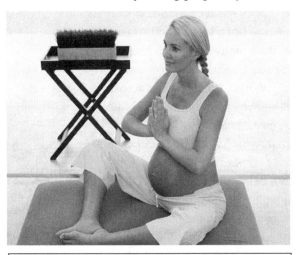

Find a regular time and a comfortable rhythm, and give it priority. You may find walking a simple and pleasant exercise during pregnancy. Or perhaps you enjoy swimming, dancing, or yoga. Let your body guide your choices. Do what feels right without pushing yourself to extremes.

A good rule of thumb is to avoid any movement that causes

Yoga, an ancient form of exercise that includes breath control, meditation, and body postures, has become popular among pregnant women. It's easy to understand why: Many yoga exercises include movements that open the pelvis. Yoga also teaches rhythmic breathing, concentration, stamina building, and relaxation. Some women who do yoga report improved physical coordination and more balanced emotions.

pain or excessive strain. (For more detailed guidelines on exercise during pregnancy, visit http://www.marchofdimes.com and search for the keyword *exercise*.)

Thomas Moore writes in *The Re-Enchantment of Everyday Life*, "It's difficult to imagine being busy and enchanted at the same time. Enchantment invites us to pause and be arrested by whatever is before us; instead of doing something, something is done to us."

We think pregnancy should be a time of enchantment. It's a time to pause, to step away from your crowded agenda, and to surrender to the delight and mystery of what is growing within you. This is a powerful and amazing thing that you and your baby are accomplishing, a dance unlike any other in the human experience.

Love Your Blooming Body

Midwife Ina May Gaskin encourages you to spend your pregnancy "loving your uterus and your body. I mean this literally. Positive energy makes a good birth outcome more likely, so go for it."[4] Early pregnancy is a great time to fall in love with your body and cheer its growth into a beautiful new shape.

Maternity clothing designers have recently begun to accentuate the beauty of a pregnant women's body. Suddenly the world is taking note of a beautiful woman standing at a crosswalk, her hands spread lovingly over her pregnant belly, wearing a clingy dress or playful pants and a shirt that accentuates, rather than hides, her shape. Thanks to modern maternity fashions and all the expectant mothers who've stepped out of their homes and into the public eye, today the pregnant body is widely perceived as a thing of beauty.

Happily watching yourself gain weight during pregnancy may be hard, but try to get used to it. Remembering *why* you're gaining weight may help: Your pregnant body is carrying not only a growing baby, but a growing placenta, amniotic fluid, increased blood volume, and growing breasts and uterus. Your body is also storing the fat needed to make the perfect food for your baby—your breast milk.

Remember this, too: A woman's good design includes a postpartum weight-loss mechanism. The months you devote to nourishing your baby with your own milk will burn off some of the fat your body stored protectively during your pregnancy. And as the active mother of a demanding newborn, you'll also sweat off some of the extra fluids your body needed in pregnancy. Pregnancy weight gain is nothing to fear. It's nature's way, and it results in a beautiful you and a healthy baby.

Make Changes for the Better

Consider whether any of the following changes might make sense in the early months of your pregnancy:

- **Changes in your schedule**: Are you striking a good balance between working and stopping work, between exercise and rest?
- **Changes in your diet**: Are you getting enough protein, fiber, iron, folic acid, and calcium? (For more on pregnancy nutrition, see page 66 or visit http://www.4woman.gov/faq/preg-nutr.htm.) Proper nutrition is important not only for your baby, but also for you. It protects against a wide array of potential problems, from maternal nutrient depletion to low birth weight. Good food for your pregnant body needn't be expensive or out of the ordinary—just wholesome and nutrient-rich. You choose what, when, and how much to eat, and try to make your choices as healthy and as balanced as possible. If you find it difficult to eat because of nausea, don't panic. Simply eat as well and as often as you can—your baby will make the most of whatever you're able to keep down. There is absolutely no evidence that either salt or calories should be restricted during pregnancy.
- **Changes in what you drink**: Are you drinking enough water? During pregnancy you need plenty of water to support your increased blood volume and your baby's amniotic fluid. Water can also help with problems like constipation, headache, nausea, muscle cramps, dry hair and skin, low energy, and much more. Drink when you're thirsty, and drink enough to satisfy your thirst. Although in the United States many doctors recommend that women drink no alcohol or caffeine at all while pregnant, there's no

research supporting total abstinence. In fact, research shows that mild caffeine consumption (one to two cups of coffee per day) is safe.[5] And *A Guide to Effective Care in Pregnancy and Childbirth* (see Appendix A) says "prohibition of all alcohol intake during pregnancy" is "not likely to be beneficial," but that "advice to avoid excessive alcohol consumption" is "likely to be beneficial."[6]

- **Changes in your habits**: Do you smoke or use street drugs? Smoking during pregnancy may not only harm your health, it may also lead to serious health problems in your baby. The risk of premature birth and low birth weight is nearly doubled for the baby of a smoking woman, and that baby inherits a higher risk of health problems. Smoking has also been linked with several birth defects. Here's the good news: Stopping or substantially reducing your smoking and staying away from secondhand smoke can greatly improve your odds of having a healthy pregnancy and a healthy baby. Street drugs, too, can be harmful to your baby's health and growth. The placenta allows most drugs (street drugs and pharmaceuticals) to reach your baby's bloodstream. Drugs like cocaine and heroin can cause premature labor, as well as addiction, stunted growth, and behavioral and emotional problems in your baby. It's extremely important to get help if you can't stop yourself.

> Many programs are available to help you stop smoking. The March of Dimes provides a practical, helpful "Tips to Quit" checklist and links to other smoking cessation organizations at its website (http://www.marchofdimes.com). While you're trying to quit, stay away from places and activities that tempt you to smoke or that might expose you to secondhand smoke. And don't get discouraged if you can't quit cold turkey right away. Cut back as much as you can, and find someone who will support your efforts.

- **Changes in your planning**: Are you making informed choices about your care and your baby's birth, or are you simply "going with the program"? Remember: Choices that are made for you or happen by default really aren't choices. You're more likely to be satisfied with your journey to motherhood if you educate yourself and are actively involved in decision making about pregnancy and birth.

Try to make changes during your pregnancy with confidence, not anxiety. Misinformation abounds in the media, old wives' tales, and on the internet, spawning a growing amount of unnecessary fear about foods, procedures, and activities that might threaten fetal health. How can you navigate this churning river of anxiety? Remember that much of the information is hearsay—it's incomplete, out-of-context, or not evidence-based. Get the full facts. (See Chapter 11 for tips and resources.) Make any changes in your lifestyle sensibly and positively, not anxiously and gullibly.

Find Good Prenatal Care

For most women pregnancy and birth require no medical intervention of any kind, but it *is* important to have good prenatal care. Good prenatal care should help you move through pregnancy healthy and confident and help you prepare for the safe, healthy birth of your baby.

Your caregiver and birth site can dramatically influence how your pregnancy and birth go, so choose carefully. It isn't critical to see a caregiver the minute you suspect you're pregnant—unless you have a preexisting medical condition like diabetes or heart disease that adds risk to your pregnancy, you suspect you have a sexually transmitted disease or other infection, or you have bleeding, pain, or severe vomiting. Otherwise you have time, and you should take that time to think about the kind of prenatal care and birth you'd like and to find a caregiver and birth site that suit you.

Choosing a Caregiver and Birth Site

It is your choice. You can do what you think is best. You don't have to agree. There is no right answer. You can take more time to decide. It's okay to follow your instincts. You can say no and still be respected.
—Alessandra Godinho

INFORMED CHOICE

Is "What Is" What's Best for You?

There's an old story about a young woman who always cut off the end of a ham before putting it her roasting pan. She'd grown up watching her mother prepare ham exactly the same way. One afternoon while she made dinner for her visiting parents, her mother watched her slice off the end of the ham. When the mother asked, "Why do you do that?" the daughter replied, "Well, it's what you always did. It's how ham should be prepared." The mother smiled and replied, "I did that because back then my only roasting pan was too small to hold a whole ham."

Like the daughter who never asked about her mother's roasting method, many women don't question modern American birth practices. They assume that what is must be what's best. There must be a good reason why so many doctors require routine ultrasounds during pregnancy. Or why so many labors are induced. Or why so many women have epidurals.

It's easy to forget that just a few decades ago, hospitals routinely used practices that we now know are useless or even harmful. They banned partners from delivery rooms. Women received enemas at the onset of labor. Newborns were suspended upside down by their feet and smacked on their little bottoms. Women got injections after birth to prevent their breasts from making milk. These practices ended because women asked questions and challenged assumptions. Women's informed choices changed the status quo.

You have a wonderful opportunity before you to make informed choices about your body and your baby's birth. Remember that these are *your* choices, not your caregiver's, not your relatives' or friends', not the hospital's or clinic's or medical textbook's. Look beyond what is—what modern obstetrics and culture dictate—and you may discover better options for you and yours. You can make your pregnancy an empowering time of learning, discerning, and choosing as you plan for your baby's arrival.

Gathering and Analyzing Information

We live in a time when lots of information (both accurate and inaccurate) on just about any subject is readily available. Technology has increased our access not only to information, but also to goods and services—simultaneously widening and narrowing our everyday choices. For example, you can have a home entertainment system that offers hundreds of viewing options, but find that none of them is worth watching. You may be able to find exotic fruits from all over the globe in your neighborhood supermarket, but not a locally grown apple.

The same paradox exists in the realm of childbirth. In the United States pregnant women have the right to make informed choices about their maternity care. (For more on the rights of childbearing women, see Appendix C.) They're legally entitled to full and clear information from their caregivers about the benefits and risks of maternity care practices. But many don't get that crucial information.[1] And those who search for it on their own face the daunting task of distinguishing obstetric myth from fact.

To make matters worse, our medicalized culture bombards us with both subtle and direct messages that make it very hard to think independently about pregnancy and birth. Watch TV programs about birth, and you're bound to see a lot of dramatic hospital scenes. Open any mainstream pregnancy or parenting magazine, and you'll see page after page of formula ads. And then there are all the individual voices joining the din. As your pregnancy progresses, more and more people will talk to you about their pregnancies and births. As you listen to all these messages and stories and recommendations—which may contradict each other or what you're reading in this book—you may wonder what really is best for you and your baby.

Here are a couple of ideas to help you analyze all the information you're gathering:

- *In the media, hospitals and doctors generally take center stage in stories about birth, while mothers play supporting roles. Does this type of role suit you?* It happens in real life, too. If you've ever had a routine medical exam, you've probably found yourself perched on an examination table, shivering in a flimsy backless gown as staff swept in and out of the room wearing lab coats or scrubs and official ID tags. It's common to feel vulnerable, awkward, and out of place in moments like these, and such feelings can diminish your power to question a professional's opinion or to consider all the factors that contribute to making the best possible healthcare decision for you. Many a pregnant woman's labor and birth decisions are made by others, long before she writes a birth plan or arrives at the hospital—as though it's all from a generic script. Considering that you are *you*, not a generic patient, would you prefer to write your own script?

- *How did the stories you're hearing come about? How did the tellers of these stories arrive at—or forfeit—their choices?* Did they make informed choices or "go with the program"? Does their information agree or conflict with the information you've gathered? Were they pleased with their outcomes? Would those outcomes please you? If you respectfully ask for more details and compare what you hear with your own values and knowledge, you're likely to get a fuller picture and wind up better equipped to make your own choices.

MYTHS ABOUT CAREGIVERS AND BIRTH SITES

Your choice of a caregiver and birth site (the two are usually linked) is one of the most important decisions you'll make during your pregnancy. It will profoundly influence the path of your pregnancy, birth, and early mothering.

Because women typically make this decision early in pregnancy, they rarely have enough time to make a truly informed decision. Instead, women often choose their

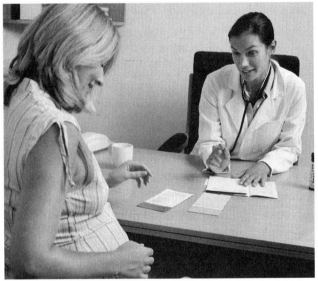

caregivers and birth sites based on convenience or on misinformation they've picked up before becoming pregnant. We urge you to take your time, to deliberately gather and scrutinize information. To help you get started, let's first dispel some widespread myths about maternity care.

Myth 1:
Pregnancy and childbirth are terribly risky.
Fact: Having a baby is a normal, natural, healthy event.
The World Health Organization (WHO) believes that 85 to 95 percent of pregnancies can be expected to go perfectly.[2] Most women enter pregnancy in good health, and this is a strong foundation for a healthy pregnancy.

Could you encounter trouble in pregnancy and labor? Yes. Should you expect it? No. Pregnancy and birth are perfectly designed by nature and are safer now than ever before—*not* because they're managed by doctors and hospitals but because women are healthier going into pregnancy and birth, because hygiene is better, and because antibiotics are widely available.

If a healthy pregnant woman lets nature take its course, her baby and her body are well protected.

Of course, some pregnancies and births are riskier. Smoking, substance abuse, and physical and psychological stress can harm both women and their babies. But these are lifestyle issues, not problems that can be prevented or fixed by medicine. Only a small percentage of women enter pregnancy with preexisting health problems (such as diabetes) or develop complications during pregnancy or birth (such as pregnancy-induced hypertension). It is for these women that medical intervention makes pregnancy and birth safer.[3]

Myth 2:
Birth is safest in a hospital with a doctor.
Fact: For most women, birth at home or at a birth center is as safe as—or safer than—at a hospital.
You may hear that in order to ensure your safety, you should see a doctor for prenatal care and give birth in a hospital—preferably one with a neonatal intensive care unit (NICU). This better-safe-than-sorry myth has been evolving for about one hundred years.

In the early 1900s there was deep concern about the maternal mortality rate; many women were dying after birth of puerperal fever. Doctors argued that poorly trained midwives contributed to this problem and insisted that doctors provided safer care. Many years later research showed that women who had been attended by doctors were *more* likely to die from puerperal fever because doctors weren't washing their hands well enough at births. Midwifery care had actually been *safer* for women.[4]

This is an example of an iatrogenic problem (a problem caused by caregivers). Iatrogenic obstetric problems have played out over and over in the years since then. Here's one modern example: Many doctors believe that continuous electronic fetal monitoring (EFM) makes labor safer for babies, so they do it routinely. However, research shows that routine continuous EFM results in no fewer babies who have problems or die[5] but more mothers who end up with cesareans.[6] So EFM makes birth riskier for mothers with no benefit for babies.

Continuous EFM is just one of many routine interventions that disrupt and create problems in otherwise normal labors and births. The medical attitude of expecting trouble, and the hospital policies that support this attitude, prevent women from giving birth easily and safely in the typical hospital and contribute to the alarming U.S. cesarean rates. Cesarean surgery increases risks for both mother and baby.[7]

In a very small percentage of pregnancies and births, complications like preexisting diabetes or heart disease, prematurity, or fetal distress during labor *should* be managed in a hospital by a doctor. But for most women, birth outside the hospital is as safe as—or safer than—hospital birth.[8]

Myth 3:
Giving birth outside a hospital or with a midwife means suffering needlessly.

Fact: There are many ways to find comfort in labor without drugs, and this search for comfort helps move labor along. Pain serves an important purpose in labor, but that purpose *isn't* maternal suffering. On the contrary: Its purpose is to compel mothers to actively seek comfort.

When allowed and encouraged to, a woman will naturally move, moan, sway, change her breathing pattern, and rock to cope with contractions, eventually finding the right rhythm for her unique needs. Such active comfort-seeking helps her baby rotate and descend and helps prevent her labor from stalling. As her contractions get stronger, her body releases endorphins—nature's narcotic—to ease her pain.

Comfort methods like activity and rest, eating and drinking, showering and bathing, receiving continuous emotional and physical support,

But what if you really *need* medication? Most midwives can prescribe medications, but they are more likely to encourage and provide for non-drug pain strategies than physicians are. Hospital midwives encourage you not to depend entirely on the epidural for pain relief, because epidurals change the normal process of labor and lead to a cascade of interventions (required to ensure that you and your baby are safe).[9] Outside the hospital there are many more options for finding comfort in labor. But, because of the medical risks of epidural and other pain medications, you will need to be in a hospital if you require or desire them.

massage, relaxation, and applying heat and cold are more available to women who give birth outside the hospital and/or are attended by midwives. In hospital births, often the only pain relief available is a drug—typically an epidural. Simple comfort measures are frequently prohibited by staff who don't understand the purpose or the value of natural comfort-seeking. Women are expected to lie quietly in bed, attached to monitors and intravenous (IV) lines, with strict limits on the number of people who can stay with and support them. Without the freedom to use a wide variety of comfort measures in labor, it's no surprise that more than 90 percent of women in some hospitals choose an epidural!

Myth 4:
Choosing midwifery care is an all-or-nothing decision.
Fact: A good midwife is a skilled member of a caregiving team.
Many women worry that if they choose midwifery care or non-hospital birth, they'll be in big trouble—with no options—if problems arise. They assume that midwives can't handle crises and reason that if there's any chance of labor complications, they'd better be in a hospital.

This line of thinking springs from inadequate understanding of the training and role of midwives. Most midwives in the U.S. today are certified nurse-midwives (CNMs). A CNM has advanced training (often a master's degree) beyond her nursing degree and has passed a rigorous certification exam. Two other types of nationally recognized midwife credentials are CM (certified midwife) and CPM (certified professional midwife). Neither is a nurse, but both are well-trained, knowledgeable, certified professionals.

All three types of certified midwives are carefully trained to provide primary care for healthy women as part of a maternity healthcare team. Their expertise is in normal pregnancy and birth. Because they're trained to recognize what is normal and natural—and because they practice based on the evidence that shows birth usually goes best without interference—their care is more likely to keep pregnancy, labor, and birth normal.

Midwives collaborate with obstetricians, who are specialists in managing pregnancy and childbirth complications. If a woman develops a health problem or requires surgery, her midwife will refer her to a doctor. All certified and licensed midwives have physician backup (doctors on call who have agreed to treat or consult with their patients who develop unexpected medical needs) and can admit women to hospitals if necessary.

Furthermore, midwives are qualified to manage many problems and emergencies. They can administer oxygen, prescribe medication including antibiotics (although this varies from state to state), start IV fluids, repair tears, and perform both adult and infant cardiopulmonary resuscitation (CPR).

Choosing a midwife and/or a non-hospital birth is a choice that changes if circumstances change. Midwives provide primary care, collaborating with doctors if needed, using guidelines approved by both midwives and obstetricians. In the countries where this model is the norm, there are fewer medical interventions and fewer deaths of mothers and babies than in the U.S.[10]

CHOOSING A CAREGIVER WHO SUPPORTS NORMAL BIRTH

What's It Like to Use a Midwife?

The hallmark of midwifery is a strong belief in the natural process of childbearing. A good midwife patiently observes, teaches, and supports you throughout your pregnancy and birth. By doing so, she helps prevent problems. However, she can quickly and accurately identify complications and call in her physician backup if necessary. She is vigilant but doesn't expect trouble. This above all defines the difference between midwifery and obstetric care.

A midwife typically has more time than a doctor has to offer patient, supportive care—not only because she cares for low-risk pregnancies, but also because her goals are different. She emphasizes staying healthy, reducing stress, building confidence, and enjoying your pregnancy. She presents prenatal testing as an option, not an unquestioned routine, and encourages you to think about what you'd do with the information.

A midwife will provide continuous hands-on help during your labor and birth and will intervene only when necessary, not routinely. She'll let your labor start, progress, and end on its own. She'll encourage you to eat, drink, and move about freely. All these practices help reduce your risk of birth injury, trauma, and cesarean surgery.[11] Industrialized countries where midwives are the primary maternity caregivers for healthy women have lower perinatal mortality rates and lower cesarean rates than the U.S.[12]

Only 10 percent of U.S. births are attended by midwives, but according to *Listening to Mothers* (a 2002 survey report on American women's childbearing experiences), women with midwives are the most satisfied with their births.[13] Approximately one in ten midwife-attended births (one percent of births in the U.S.) is a home birth. (Almost all U.S. home births are attended by midwives—usually CPMs or CMs.) The other nine percent happen in hospitals or birth centers (with CNMs).

Today there's a growing concern that some midwives are practicing like obstetricians—that they're expecting trouble in pregnancy and birth and are acting accordingly. If

"When people ask me why I have a midwife, I can only respond that not every situation needs to be medicalized. Here's what I mean: I arrived at Brigham and Women's Hospital fully dilated. While the admissions staff tried to get me to do paperwork, I lay stretched out on the floor trying to get into my hypno-birthing relaxation mode. The staff hit a code blue because they had no idea what I was doing; they thought something was wrong. As everyone scrambled around me, I heard a voice down the hall. It was Biddy, our midwife. I felt calm and relaxed the moment I heard her voice and felt her touch. She pressed my head into her chest and hugged me. There was no reason to think anything was wrong. I was in labor, the most natural process in the world! I just needed people to let me do the work that my body and my baby knew how to do. That's exactly what Biddy did. During Ryan's birth Biddy and Dennis supported me, but they let me do what I knew how to do. Ryan was born forty-five minutes later—a healthy little boy with gorgeous eyes and beautiful red hair. As I await the birth of our second child, I'm free of worry and fear. Biddy has taught me to trust myself and my baby."
—Michelle

you want to keep your birth as natural as possible, be wary of a midwife who's controlling and prescriptive, who frightens you, who's content to go along with restrictive hospital policies, who pressures you into prenatal testing, or who won't stay with you throughout your labor. You probably won't be happy with her.

What's It Like to Have an Obstetrician as a Primary Caregiver?

Obstetric training focuses on caring for women with complications or those who are at high risk for complications, so it's no surprise that most obstetricians view pregnancy as an illness and birth as fraught with danger. Obstetric prenatal care tends to focus on screening for abnormalities, and childbirth under obstetric care is usually closely monitored and controlled.[14] Obstetricians diagnose problems based on narrow definitions of normalcy. As a result, pregnancy and childbirth transform from a normal, natural process to an intervention-intensive medical event.

If you have complications, you truly do need an obstetrician's expertise for at least part of your maternity care. But if you're healthy and your pregnancy is low-risk (as is the case 85 to 95 percent of the time), you may not receive the most appropriate care in a typical obstetric practice.[15] After a long career of research, practice, and teaching in public health, epidemiologist and midwife Judith Rooks has concluded that in too many obstetric practices, "the level of surveillance and intervention well exceeds the elements of necessary care."[16] This may seem harmless, but an attitude of expecting trouble may actually increase your risk and probably will increase your fear.

Most obstetricians routinely order prenatal tests like ultrasound, alpha-fetoprotein screening, and gestational diabetes screening. But many women don't receive full information about the accuracy of tests or the information that tests can and can't provide. And women are often pressured if they express misgivings or refuse prenatal testing. During labor, an obstetrician is likely to use routine interventions (like continuous EFM and IV lines), and you can expect your labor to be moved along quickly. And ironically, though obstetricians tend to expect trouble, an obstetrician probably won't stay with you throughout labor.

Research suggests that for all these reasons, there are few, if any, benefits of obstetric care for healthy, low-risk pregnancies. *A Guide to Effective Care in Pregnancy and Childbirth* summarizes the evidence: "It is inherently unwise, and perhaps unsafe, for women with normal pregnancies to be cared for by obstetric specialists."[17]

Even if you've been pleased with an ob-gyn's (obstetrician-gynecologist's) wellness care, you may not be equally pleased with his or her maternity care. Your needs change when you become pregnant, so it's important that you ask questions. For example:

- What prenatal testing is done routinely?
- What labor practices are used routinely?
- What are your doctor's rates of inductions, episiotomies (see page 153), instrument deliveries, and cesareans?
- What does he or she think about doulas?
- Does he or she seem to have more confidence in interventions than your ability to give birth?

Veteran midwife Ina May Gaskin advises, "If any of your questions provokes resentment, sarcasm, hostility, scare tactics, or vague or patronizing answers, keep shopping."[18] We add: Beware of doctors who simply tell you what you want to hear, who kindly brush aside your questions to get past them and move on to a more comfortable discussion.

What about a female obstetrician? Many women believe that female doctors are likely to practice more compassionately. This isn't a safe assumption. Though a woman may have firsthand experience of birth or may have a more sensitive manner, all obstetricians—regardless of gender—are trained to view birth as a medical event.

How Does a Doctor-Midwife Practice Work?

In a doctor-midwife partnership, an obstetrician employs a midwife to care for healthy, low-risk women, and the doctor cares for those who have complications or are at high risk for problems. The midwife and doctor work as a team to attend births—usually in hospitals, but sometimes in birth centers or homes.

A doctor-midwife practice isn't always the best of both worlds. If the midwife covers only office visits while the doctor manages births, or if the practice routinely uses labor interventions like continuous EFM or restrictions on eating and drinking, this might indicate a belief that birth is a medical event, not a natural process.

A practice like this can work very well, though. Biddy Fein directs a large midwifery service attending births at Boston's Brigham and Women's Hospital, one of the biggest and most respected maternity hospitals in the U.S. She says, "At Brigham and Women's we have a wonderful collaboration with the physicians. They take care of the women with medical problems, but we continue to see these women. We provide the care that ensures they will be confident, be able to work with their labors, be supported—none of these things goes out the window just because they have medical problems. These women need midwives even more."[19] We agree.

What's It Like to Have Maternity Care with a Family Doctor?

Family doctors provide comprehensive medical care with emphasis on the family unit. They used to provide a great deal of obstetric care in the U.S., especially in rural areas. (They still do in some areas.) Though all family doctors have some obstetric training, only about 30 percent include obstetrics in their practice. The cost of malpractice insurance, the fear of lawsuits, and the demands of attending births around the clock have all contributed to this decline.[20]

Many family doctors are concerned about the current level of routine obstetric intervention. The American Academy of Family Physicians (AAFP) encourages its members "to develop a style of obstetrical practice that recognizes that most pregnancies require no specific 'medical' intervention," and to forge "closer ties with the growing number of well-trained midwives." [21]

Some family doctors provide care that's very similar to typical obstetric care, while others provide care that's more like midwifery. Find out the style of a particular family doctor by asking questions. (See page 49.)

Making Your Choice

The best caregiver for you is the one who helps you feel the most confident and supported as you journey through pregnancy, labor, and birth. Whether you choose an obstetrician, a family doctor, or a midwife, it's important that he or she listen to you, respect your ideas and questions, and encourage you to make truly informed decisions.

Pay attention to your gut feelings. Be cautious about recommendations from friends and family. What's important to others may not be what's important to you. You may also be finding that your own priorities in pregnancy and birth are changing.

"With my first baby, I'm sure I would have chosen the path that most women choose today—an obstetrician and a medically managed labor—if not for my friend Maureen. When her first baby was born a few years before mine, she used a CNM and had an unmedicated, low-tech birth. Maureen had fifty-six hours of back labor with this wonderful nine-pound girl, and she came away from it seeming so powerful and proud, not victimized and complaining like most other women I knew. She spoke about everything she did as if it were the normal way that women gave birth. She said labor was hard, but she was so high and felt so fine after her baby was born that I knew when I had my baby I would try to do it the same way. As I think about it now, I realize this is just what women did before the last few generations became so terrified of birth. I learned from a woman who had walked the path before me, and I felt confident."

—Allison

CHOOSING A SITE THAT SUPPORTS NORMAL BIRTH

You may choose to have your baby at home, at a birth center (freestanding or within a hospital), or at a hospital. These environments are very different and will powerfully influence how your labor and birth progress. Your choice also shapes the preparation you must do to ensure that you'll feel confident and supported during labor. This choice will also influence what happens to you and your baby after the birth.

Questions to Ask

The Coalition for Improving Maternity Services (CIMS) firmly believes in a woman's right to choose how she'll give birth. (For more information on CIMS, see page 20 and

Appendix B.) CIMS encourages you to think ahead about care for you and your baby at the time of birth. It calls care that's healthier for mothers and babies "mother-friendly." CIMS suggests that when you're investigating birth sites, you should ask the following questions to learn more about your options at each site and to help you choose the site that's most likely to support normal birth.[22]

- **Who can be with me during labor and birth?** Some support people you may want are your baby's father, your partner (if he or she isn't your baby's father), your children, other family members, friends, a doula, and/or a midwife. Can you have all, some, or none of these people with you?

- **What happens during normal labor?** You should be able to get statistics on every part of the birth process at the site. For example, how often is labor induced? What, if anything, is done to speed up labor and birth? How many cesareans are performed per year?

- **How does this site accommodate differences in culture and belief?** Families have widely varying values and customs regarding issues like who may witness a birth, ceremonies or rituals during labor or after birth, symbolic or spiritual objects present in the room, and so on.

- **Can I walk and change positions during labor and pushing?** Being allowed to move about as you wish and to choose your position for pushing is important for your comfort and confidence.

- **What birth practices are considered normal and used routinely?** Keep an eye out for common interventions, like those listed below, that have been proven ineffective or harmful for mothers or babies. (For more information, see Chapter 8, pages 114–120, and Appendix A, pages 238–241.)
    - Continuous EFM that restricts a mother's mobility: Intermittent EFM or auscultation (listening to the baby's heart rate) provides equally useful information with less chance of misreading a printout and better mobility for the mother.
    - Prohibiting or restricting food and drink during labor: This is an old practice that many hospitals have

abandoned because research shows women need energy and hydration to do the hard work of labor.

- Shaving a mother's pubic hair or giving her an enema: These, too, are archaic practices shown to provide absolutely no benefits to a laboring woman.

- Insertion of an IV needle: Women are told that this provides quicker access to their bloodstream in case of emergency. But needles and IV lines can restrict mobility, and the sight and feel of them can increase stress.

- **Besides drugs, how will you help me deal with labor pain?** In most cases, non-drug coping methods give mothers more confidence and control and are safer for mothers and babies. Does the site offer a variety of methods to help you stay as comfortable as possible in labor? (Some non-drug comfort measures are helping you change positions, a warm bath or shower, massage, and providing a birth ball for rest and movement.) Or is the site inflexible, giving mothers no choice but to depend on medication for pain relief?

- **How will you help me with breastfeeding?** The WHO has made breastfeeding a priority in its policies for improving the health of babies around the world. In accordance with the WHO, a birth site should be telling all its maternity patients about the importance of breast-feeding, and it should have policies in place to ensure that babies nurse during the first hour of life and receive only breast milk, unless there's a valid medical reason a baby can't. Mothers should be encouraged to feed their babies on demand. There should always be staff available who know how to help mothers with breastfeeding, and mothers should be given the name of a person or group to contact for support and information. A birth site should not give away free samples of baby formula.

More about Hospital Birth

Hospitals are designed to deal with illness. If you're among the 85 to 95 percent of pregnant women who are healthy and low-risk, you don't need to give birth in a hospital. But if you have preexisting health problems or develop serious complications during your pregnancy, labor, or birth, the hospital is exactly where you should be.

Some hospitals have worked hard to provide more homelike birthing rooms and to reduce the number of rules that hinder normal birth, but you can still expect to have less freedom at a hospital than you would at home or at a birth center. A homelike birth unit doesn't translate into a homelike birth. Common hospital interventions like IV use, eating and drinking restrictions, and continuous EFM can make it harder to work actively with your labor. If you do choose to give birth in a hospital, you'll need a birth plan that helps you avoid or limit the negative effects of hospital policies. (See Chapter 10.)

Most women look forward to having help from a labor and delivery nurse in the hospital and expect her to be a calm, supportive presence throughout labor.[23] Research suggests that this is an unrealistic expectation. In today's high-tech birth culture, a labor and delivery nurse spends most of her time monitoring IV fluid intake, EFM, and induction; assisting at cesareans; and taking care of women with serious problems.[24] Although most labor nurses would *like* to stay at your side, they simply don't have the time.

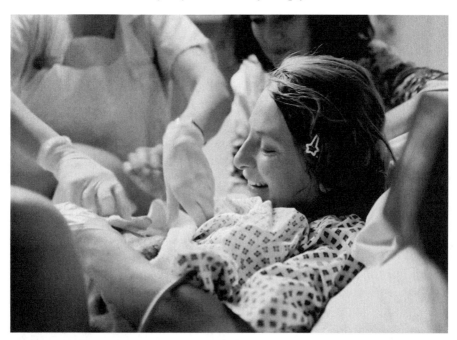

"My spirits were high as the nurse announced that I was three centimeters dilated and 100 percent effaced. My doctor told me that if my labor didn't progress throughout the night, I would be induced in the morning. I wasn't worried; I had a strong feeling I'd give birth by then. I trusted my body and ignored all the horrendous stories of pain and cesareans, reminding myself of all the women who have gone through this life-changing, thrilling event.

The nurses didn't interfere much. Justin and I knew it was important for me to change positions and use the bathroom every hour, and that helped my contractions grow stronger. Lying on my back was uncomfortable, so I mostly labored on my sides, leaning against Justin, or sitting in the shower. We all dozed on and off.

As my contractions grew stronger, Justin and Chris, my doula, massaged me. I visualized being at the ocean, with waves of contractions washing over me, and the pain was manageable. I moved into the shower, and Justin stayed with me, telling me I was doing a wonderful job. I was relieved at how smoothly my labor had progressed and never considered pain meds, even when a nurse asked if I wanted any.

As my contractions began to double-peak, I vomited. I recognized this sign of transition and was excited to be closer to meeting my baby. I knew my body was working to get my baby safely out, and I remembered that this stage wouldn't last long. I kept thinking, 'After this contraction, there'll be one less I have to conquer.'

Then came the urge to push. I let my body tell me what to do. I decided the toilet would be most comfortable to push on, and Justin and Chris joined me there, massaging, comforting, and encouraging me. When the doctor came in to check me and said I could start pushing, he didn't realize I'd already been pushing for a half-hour.

I got on my hands and knees, and with lots more encouragement, pushing, and rocking, my son Dylan Alan was born on Sunday morning. He was so beautiful, with amazing cries, a full head of hair, and such a tiny face. He had a wonderful Apgar score, but because he was premature, I could hold him for only a moment before he was taken to the NICU. Justin followed him, and a kind nurse kept me informed about his condition.

After I was discharged, Dylan stayed in the hospital for a week and I became a boarder. He needed some time and help learning to breastfeed. But now he's happy and thriving on my milk. Although my birth didn't go exactly according to plan, I have good memories of it. I remember the visualizing I did during labor. Dylan's name means 'of the sea.' He is calm and flexible—an amazing, bright, and beautiful little boy. He is a gift, and it was a good birth."

—Claire

Because of this, if you choose a hospital birth, you'll need to supply your own continuous labor support. Consider hiring a doula in addition to having support from your partner, family, and/or friends. The presence of an experienced, knowledgeable, reassuring woman can help you remain confident during labor and work effectively with your contractions. A doula can also help your other support people help you. A doula may even help you feel more comfortable about staying at home for most of your labor. Research suggests that the longer you're in the hospital and the more interventions you have, the less satisfied with your birth you're likely to be.[25]

Though normal birth is more challenging in a hospital, it's definitely possible with good planning and a confident attitude. Claire's story (see page 55) is a wonderful example of normal birth in a hospital. She had personal and professional support, her obstetrician didn't interfere in the natural process, and in spite of her baby's prematurity, Claire was encouraged to breastfeed him.

More about Birth outside a Hospital

Most women who choose hospital birth do so because they believe that's the safest place to have a baby, "in case something goes wrong." Most health professionals believe this, too. This opinion is based on observing the poor outcomes of unplanned non-hospital births.[26] A closer look at the research tells the real story.

A number of studies compare hospital births and planned non-hospital births. *Planned* non-hospital births are safe. *A Guide to Effective Care in Pregnancy and Childbirth* concludes that "women who have no factors that contraindicate a home birth, and who prefer a planned, attended home birth with facilities for prompt transfer to hospital if necessary, should not be advised against it"[27] Of all the women surveyed for *Listening to Mothers*, only those who gave birth outside hospitals reported receiving all six care practices that support normal birth (see page 4).[28]

Birth at a Birth Center

A birth center may be either freestanding or located within a hospital. Birth centers provide many of the comforts of home plus a number of comforts that may not be available at home, like whirlpool tubs. At some birth centers, a variety of pain medications

> To find a birth center near you, call the National Association of Childbearing Centers (NACC) at 215-234-8068 or visit NACC's website at http://www.birthcenters.org.

are available. Emergency equipment for mother and baby are always available. Every birth center has physician backup and a system for hospital transfer if complications arise.

The philosophy of a good birth center is that birth is a normal, natural, healthy process and that women have an inherent ability to give birth. A good birth center has no routine interventions and gives women freedom to respond to their contractions in any way that seems right. Be wary of a facility that calls itself a birth center but doesn't differ in philosophy or policy from the standard hospital.

Birth centers are usually staffed by midwives, but some doctors attend births in this setting. Although many women who choose birth centers hire doulas, they also receive continuous labor support from the nurses on staff. This is possible because with fewer restrictive rules, the nurses' time isn't consumed with managing medical interventions and complications. Typically women return home several hours after giving birth at a birth center.

> "My daughter Mary had her first child at a hospital birth center. Mary labored for twelve hours, walking the quiet, carpeted halls, moving from birth ball to tub. Her midwife rocked in the corner, knitting patiently but watchfully. Her nurse waited quietly and patiently, too. Mary worked very hard, occasionally teetering on the edge of despair, but always supported and encouraged by her husband and me. After a few frantic contractions in the whirlpool, finally baby Nora rotated, descending at great speed. After her birth, Nora snuggled in the big bed with her mommy and daddy. Within thirty minutes the birthing room transformed into a party room. Trays of lasagna and salad arrived. Champagne corks popped. Two ecstatic families toasted Nora's birth and Mary's hard work. All the while, Nora nursed and slept in Mary's arms.
>
> Mary had her second child at the same birth center two years later. This time, she arrived shortly after dawn, labored briefly in the tub, and gave birth quickly. Big sister Nora arrived soon after the birth, and several hours later everyone went home. The whole process—from labor starting to homecoming—took six hours. The party happened at home, with Mary and baby Molly tucked into their own bed."
> —Judith

Birth at Home

The 1900s saw a dramatic shift from home birth to hospital birth, but there's growing interest in bringing birth back home. Why is this shift happening? Simply put: Research is showing that hospitals may not be the best places to have babies unless there are specific medical needs that can't be met at home.[29]

Birth is a normal, natural process, and in the vast majority of pregnancies, there's no reason to expect problems. Any problem that might arise can be identified and handled promptly at home. A skilled caregiver sees warning signs well before there's serious danger. He or she can manage most problems—by starting an IV, administering oxygen, and so on—or can consult with a doctor and move to a hospital if necessary.

The great advantage of giving birth at home is that home is where most women feel safest and most comfortable. It's where they can truly relax and be themselves. At home, it's so much easier to be undisturbed than it is at a facility full of unfamiliar people, sights, sounds, and smells. And at home, there are no hospital-borne supergerms to fear.

When you give birth at home, you don't have to worry about when to go to the hospital. You don't need to follow (or avoid) regulations that make sense in a large institution but make labor and birth more difficult. You have complete freedom to do whatever brings you comfort: curling up on your sofa, making a cup of tea, watching your favorite video, snuggling under your grandma's quilt, resting in your own bed. Your baby stays warm in your arms from the moment of birth—no whisking away for a bath, eye drops, or testing—and can nurse immediately. You choose the caregivers, family, and friends you want helping you, wear your own clothes, sleep in your own bed, eat your own food.

Is Home Birth Right for You?

The American College of Nurse-Midwives (ACNM) sees the choice of home birth as one that a woman and her midwife make together. If you'd like to have a home birth, you and your midwife should evaluate your overall health, obstetric history, nutritional status, home environment, and social support to make sure that you are low-risk (in other words, that you're very likely to have a healthy pregnancy and give birth normally with no serious problems).[30] Here are some questions to consider:

- Are you in good general health?
- Are you committed to maintaining a healthy pregnancy?
- Are you committed to birth without medication?
- Do you have an adequate social support network?
- Do you have privacy and physical and emotional safety at home?
- Are you willing to share responsibility for your maternity care?
- Do you have a midwife or doctor experienced in attending home births?
- Can your caregiver provide vigilant but low-intervention care?
- Does your caregiver have physician backup and hospital admitting privileges?
- Can you arrange for safe, quick transport to a hospital if necessary?
- Do you accept that if your circumstances change, a home birth might not be possible?

Complications that require hospital resources include substance abuse, multiple babies (usually), prematurity, fetal distress, and maternal insulin-dependent diabetes. Other conditions, like a pregnancy that goes well past its due date, can be handled in collaboration with a doctor. Clear and honest communication between a woman and her midwife are essential to determining whether home birth remains a safe choice. For more detailed information about planning a home birth, we recommend reading Sheila Kitzinger's *Birth Your Way*.[31]

"The long summer days leading up to Mary's third birth were relaxed and easy. She ordered a birth kit from the internet. Miriam, her midwife, visited weekly. Big sisters Nora and Molly waited happily for the new baby. I asked Mary, 'Do you have everything ready?' She answered, 'What's to get ready?' This baby would slide easily into the rhythm of her family's life.

Miriam visited one morning, and Mary complained of some pressure. She felt big and tired. Miriam offered to stay. No, Mary wanted to take a shower and get on with her day. Her husband, Rob, had already planned to be home, and they called me to say something might be up. It was eleven o'clock.

When I arrived, Mary, freshly showered and dressed, was pacing and shaking her arms wildly—her usual ritual for coping with hard labor. Her girls were playing happily with their aunts upstairs. At 11:35 Mary said, 'I have to push.' Miriam was still in transit. Mary rocked and swayed and changed position. I was amazed at how serene we all were. I thought, 'I wonder what the neighbors will think when they realize a baby is being born here.' Miriam swept in the door at 11:40, filled a bowl with water, opened her birth kit, and turned down the air conditioner.

Mary said, 'This really hurts. I'm not doing so good.' We quietly, firmly encouraged her. Baby Maggie (all nine and a half pounds of her) was born at 11:50 as her sisters, aunts, and grandfather raced down the stairs and into the room. Everyone piled on the bed, exclaiming over the sweet baby already nursing happily. Molly, we learned later from the photos we'd taken, birthed and nursed her doll over and over during the next hours.

This birth happened so simply. There were no interventions, no vaginal exams, no episiotomy, no suctioning, no eye drops, no vitamin K, no separation, no speeding up delivery of the placenta—nothing to distract Mary from the work of labor or the joy of holding her baby.

An hour later, Miriam weighed Maggie and helped Mary to the shower. We put fresh sheets on the bed, then we all ate lunch. As Maggie nursed, Miriam fed Mary grapes and gave her sips of Gatorade. Maggie was alert and nursed off and on for almost three hours. It was very peaceful.

Later in the afternoon, the traditional party started. Mary and Maggie were tucked into bed, alternately dozing and joining the festivities. Family and close friends ate and toasted the miracle of this baby. Life moved effortlessly on. Mary and Rob gave us a gift that day: not just their beautiful baby girl, but also the chance to see just how simple birth really is."

—Judith

A Few Tips As You Make Your Choice

The birth site you choose should be the one that makes you feel the most secure. But no matter where you give birth, a big chunk of your labor should take place at home. You'll need a plan to help labor along and to find comfort as you move through labor.

Know that the work of childbirth is usually more challenging in a hospital. Also keep in mind that an obstetrician is an "insurance policy" whether he or she is your primary caregiver or your caregiver's physician backup. Choosing non-hospital birth doesn't mean you won't need a hospital or that you can't go to a hospital. Every safe birth plan includes physician and hospital backup.

HOW WILL YOU VIEW YOUR PREGNANCY?

Marilyn Curl, a labor and delivery nurse and childbirth educator, suggests that every pregnant woman visit both a midwife and a doctor before choosing a caregiver: "Midwives care for healthy women, and physicians care for the sick. Hopefully, a comparison visit would help women decide how to view pregnancy. I think most young women today consider themselves healthy and capable, and midwives are best suited to reinforce that view."

How will you view your pregnancy? We encourage you to choose a confident outlook. Instead of anxiously attending prenatal checkups to hear from others how you're doing, why not enjoy your growing baby, discover the changing you, and let your caregiver know how you're doing? Instead of worrying about your baby's due date, why not rest in the knowledge that your body and your baby will start labor at just the right time?

No matter who your caregiver is, he or she should acknowledge that you are the expert in your pregnancy and that you already know how to do the work you need to do. Whether you choose a hospital, birth center, or home, your labor and birth should be interfered with only if it's clear that the benefits of intervention outweigh the risks.

As your pregnancy progresses and birth approaches, you may find that the choices you've made don't feel as right as they once did. Trust your instincts, and don't be afraid to change your mind. Many women—even very late in pregnancy—change doctors or change to a midwife, change hospitals or decide to have a birth center birth. None of your decisions needs to be etched in stone.

Chapter 5

MIDDLE AND LATE PREGNANCY

*The first home you have
is your body.*
—Ursula Knoki-Wilson

THE SHAPE OF THINGS IN THE MIDDLE MONTHS

In the early months of pregnancy, you learn to adjust as your body becomes home to a new little body inside you. The middle months also bring an avalanche of change for your body, but by now you're probably better at adjusting to the changes—you're more energized, sleeping better, and over your nausea. During these middle months, you could probably tackle most normal activities, just like before you were pregnant. It's almost as though your body has gotten the hang of what it's being asked to do. You and your baby have set up a nice, calm rhythm, both growing and getting ready for labor and birth in these golden, waiting months.

Physical Growth

Some of the changes you experience are physical. You may notice changes in the color of skin across your abdomen, where your flesh begins to show the effects of stretching to accommodate the growth underneath. Your breasts may be less sensitive than in prior months, and they're beginning to produce colostrum, their first milk. Stretch marks may show up there as well. Your complexion may either display its most radiant state or produce bothersome pimples. Increased blood volume and changes in hormone levels may lead to varicose veins in your legs, hemorrhoids, bleeding gums, or even nosebleeds—all normal responses from your body. Making smart, healthy choices will help, such as putting up your feet as much as possible, eating fiber-rich foods that will help with constipation, and gently brushing and flossing your teeth on a regular basis. Also, drinking plenty of liquids—especially water—will help prevent urinary tract infections and keep dry skin at bay. Wearing cotton under-clothes and loose clothing will prevent increased fluid secretions from getting trapped and leading to vaginal infections.

Although you might not yet have that cumbersome feeling that comes with late pregnancy, backaches may become a growing complaint because of the shift in posture, belly size, and body proportions. Baths, warm compresses, massages, gentle exercise, and heating pads may help with the strain. Placing pillows between your knees or propping pillows behind your back or under your belly will provide relief when you lie down. Some women find relief for their backs by getting down on all fours and slowly arching their backs up, like a stretching cat, and doing pelvic tilts. This helps shift the weight down into the muscles a bit—a pleasant change from how things rest in the upright stance.

A daily walk builds stamina and tones pelvic muscles.

It also oxygenates your body, aids in digestion and efficient calorie use, and may help you sleep better. And the gentleness of walking makes it the perfect preparation exercise for labor and birth. Taking a walk might be that daily appointment with yourself that we discussed in Chapter 3, a time for self-affirmation, relaxed breathing, and confidence building. You might also appreciate yoga as a stress release, a time for centering your busy mind, and a gentle opportunity to build stamina and confidence. Need some help learning how to do yoga? Pregnancy yoga videos are available in most public libraries, and you can enroll for classes in many communities. Many women testify to the benefits of yoga in pregnancy, especially because it can later become a technique for relaxation and centering attention in labor.

In these middle months you'll welcome the sensation of your baby's movements. You may describe the first flutterings (or quickening) you feel from your baby as bubbles popping or little fish darting about. Your baby has actually been moving about well before you were able to feel the sensation. But in these months, the baby has grown big enough to explore the little world inside you and make noticeable contact with the sides of your uterus. The baby's body grows to be up to ten inches long during this time, and the head, arms, and legs are more proportioned like a newborn's. He or she now has hair and blinking eyes. Along with all that growth comes a burst of activity. As the weeks go by, your baby will be up to all sorts of antics: kicking, sleeping, hiccupping, turning over, sucking that newly defined little thumb.

A Time for Emotional Growth, Too

These middle months bring heightened awareness of not only the physical and hormonal changes in pregnancy, but also the psychological impact of growing a baby. You may become intensely aware of all sorts of feelings, from sadness to elation, confidence to fear. Dreams may become more vivid, symbolic, or nonsensical than in prepregnancy. These dreams are opportunities for growth, for self-discovery, for facing fears, and for learning new strengths and insights.

If painful memories or unresolved issues emerge, it's best to deal with them rather than ignore or dismiss them. Seek out support from a trusted friend or family member or a support group recommended by your caregiver, childbirth educator, library, or health club. It's a time to pay close attention to your emotions, but you don't have to navigate the sometimes choppy emotional waters of pregnancy alone.

Above all, you need to keep the lines of communication open and keep relationships healthy as your body, mind, and baby change and grow. Expressing hopes, fears, and concerns; facing tough questions; and figuring out strategies for coping are abilities that will accompany you into the challenging and exciting years of parenting ahead.

NOURISHING YOUR BODY

In the middle months, your appetite increases, often with cravings for certain foods, such as things that are sour or salty. You may not necessarily crave the foods that were your favorites before pregnancy. This is a pleasurable time of answering unique food cravings and following your body's lead, but it's also an important time to make simple choices for good nutrition. Pregnant or not, you benefit from healthy eating with better overall wellness, healthier skin and hair, and more energy.

Healthy Eating

That said, eating healthy isn't always easy, and the pleasure of eating well during pregnancy can get drowned out if you try to strictly follow a detailed diet. That's because many health practitioners don't agree on just what "good nutrition" is—how much of a particular food is right or how many calories and fat grams you should consume. In a world of different cultural foods and customs, it's clear that there's no single right diet for a pregnant woman to follow.

The best thing to do is remember that good eating need not be a complex ordeal. What's most important is that you enjoy what you eat, eat when you're hungry, and stop when you're full. Beyond that, nutritionist Jill Stansbury's simple suggestion for good nutrition is "eating a rainbow of natural food colors." Healthy amounts of vitamins C and B_6, iron, calcium, folic acid, protein, fiber, and unsaturated fats naturally show up in fresh fruits and vegetables, dairy foods, fresh nuts and grains, lean meats, poultry, and fish. Here are some basic suggestions for eating well, whether or not pregnancy is in the picture:

- Choose foods high in vitamin C, which strengthens blood vessels, aids in healing, and helps the body resist infection and absorb iron. Look for brightly colored vegetables (green and red peppers, broccoli, Brussels sprouts, squash, and sweet potatoes) and fresh fruits (oranges and kiwi fruit) and juices.

- Choose foods high in B$_6$, which aids body growth, brain and immune systems, hormone regulation, and blood cell production. Look for bananas, fresh vegetables, dried beans (limas, pintos, and chickpeas), and fresh nuts and cereals.
- Choose foods high in iron, the nutrient known as the red-blood-cell builder. Iron can be absorbed more easily by your body with the help of vitamin C. Some good sources are dark molasses (stirred into a glass of milk), brewer's yeast (stirred into juice or baked into muffins), dark green leafy vegetables, prunes, raisins, and nuts.
- Choose foods high in calcium, important not only for healthy bones and teeth (yours and baby's), but also for blood clotting and muscle function. Enough calcium now will help protect your bone health during your breastfeeding months and beyond. Pay attention to dairy foods, leafy vegetables, whole grains, carrot juice, tofu, and nuts. Yogurt is a great pregnancy food, especially if it contains live acidophilus, a good bacteria found naturally in your body. More than just a calcium provider, yogurt has been found to aid digestion, promote healthy skin and bones, help balance intestinal bacteria, and keep vaginal yeast in check.
- Choose foods high in folic acid (another B vitamin), which is essential to the formation of the baby's spinal cord and brain systems, tissue growth, and cell division. Eat plenty of broccoli, spinach, and other dark green leafy vegetables, as well as dried beans and peas, asparagus, sunflower seeds, oranges, berries, whole grains (especially in breads and pastas), and fortified cereals. The U.S. Public Health Service suggests that women need to be getting more folic acid even before they get pregnant. And *A Guide to Effective Care in Pregnancy and Childbirth* recommends paying close attention to folic acid in your diet (or taking a folic acid supplement) for two months before conceiving, especially if you have a family history of neural tube defects.[1]
- Choose foods high in protein, which, second only to water, makes up most of your body's essential weight. Protein accomplishes your body's general repairs and maintenance as well as builds muscles and skin. Lean meats, poultry, fish, eggs, soy and milk products, and nuts are good sources. Vegetarians know that eating whole grains and dried beans

throughout the day, not necessarily together at the same meal, will satisfy protein needs.

- Choose "good" fats (essential fatty acids, found in fresh nuts, seeds, certain oils, and avocados) and avoid "bad" fats (animal fats and the saturated fats in processed and prepared foods). *Fat* is often the bad word of diet-speak, but healthy fats help control blood pressure and aid hormone and cell production. Unhealthy fats, on the other hands, are present in so much of what we eat, despite our body's minimum need for them. For some women, those fatty foods may cause indigestion, skin problems, and unnecessary weight gain. Read food labels and look out for hydrogenated fats or "trans fats." These are empty calorie foods that are not worth your time.

- Choose foods high in fiber, which, along with drinking plenty of water, reduces constipation brought on by increased hormones that slow down digestion. Fiber is found only in plants—fruits, vegetables, and whole grains.

- And don't forget these miscellaneous gems: Ginger is a useful herb to help with nausea and settle the stomach after birth. Peppermint might work the same way. Teas are the best vehicles for ginger and peppermint. Garlic is also your friend, boosting your body's ability to stave off infection, aiding in healing and digestion, helping rid the body of toxins, and improving the health of your intestines, heart, and skin. Garlic has been defined as a food, an herb, a medicinal plant, and more. Fresh bulbs are inexpensive, and they'll improve the taste of soup, stew, vegetables, meat, poultry, or fish.

What about Supplemental Vitamins?

Should you take supplemental prenatal vitamins? The use of vitamins dates back to 1500 B.C. Since then, science has researched the needs for and uses of vitamins and other supplements, but our understanding is far from complete. Today there's little agreement about their necessity or about what vitamins to take and in what proportion. It seems for every news bulletin announcing a breakthrough discovery about how a certain vitamin improves health, there's another one down the road announcing that we shouldn't be taking so much of that vitamin after all.

Before commercial vitamin supplements came on the market, women were able, even in less-than-ideal dietary circumstances, to birth healthy babies. While a prenatal vitamin seems good "insurance" if you're not getting enough of the right stuff naturally from your diet, no research confirms the need for routine use of them.[2] Trying to get the "right" dosage of prenatal vitamins isn't an exact science. The best thing you can do is eat a well-balanced and varied diet of fresh, unprocessed foods.

What about Fad Diets?

While pregnancy can be a time of new cravings, it shouldn't be a time for new fad diets. Specialty diets that exclude certain food categories, such as carbohydrates, do not fulfill a pregnant women's nutritional needs. For example, carbohydrates have been called "universal building blocks." They have the important job of providing energy to cells in the body, and they make up many of the essential staple foods humans rely on around the world, such as rice, potatoes, corn, and wheat. Rather than eliminate carbs altogether, choose those that convert more slowly into glucose. Choose brown rice rather than white, whole wheat rather than white bread, whole juices rather than processed fruit drinks. In other words, choosing unprocessed foods rather than refined foods will ensure a healthy, balanced diet. Diet fads come and go. Now's not the time to dally in them.

What about Lattes and Chocolate Bars?

Visit one chat room, and you'll probably see an ever-growing list of pregnancy no-nos when it comes to foods. So what are the facts about two of our favorite vices—caffeine and chocolate?

There's no agreement about how much is too much caffeine during pregnancy. While some folks preach abstinence from all caffeine, there's no evidence that moderate amounts (one to two cups of coffee per day) have any effect on your baby.[3] If you get a great deal of pleasure from of a good cup of coffee, enjoy your latte.

Now, about chocolate—there's good news from Finland. Researchers there have found that six-month-old babies born to mothers who ate chocolate during pregnancy smiled and

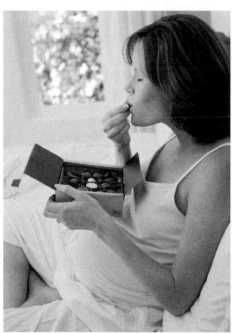

laughed more and showed milder reactions to stress than babies of mothers who abstained from chocolate. The researchers' conclusion: The chemicals in chocolate associated with positive moods might indeed pass from mother to baby during pregnancy.[4]

But What about Weight Gain?

With so much emphasis on eating, it's hard for some women not to worry about weight gain during pregnancy. But take a glance around, and you'll see that we all come in different sizes, especially during pregnancy. Even with similar diets and activity levels, women vary greatly in how much weight they gain (including how much is baby and how much is placenta and body fluids) and how their bodies carry that weight (all in front, on the sides, up high, or down low). There is no normal range of weight gain, although the American College of Obstetricians and Gynecologists (ACOG) recommends at least twenty-five to thirty-five pounds. Placing too much emphasis on pounds and a potential postpartum weight-loss struggle can lead to negative self-images.

Again, the best thing you can do is eat a healthy, balanced diet. Knowing you're eating well to nourish both you and your baby may help you feel better about your changing body. And don't forget that nature has a perfect plan for that extra fat you store during pregnancy: Nine hundred calories a day are used producing breast milk! But if negative feelings about how your body looks still overtake positive feelings about what your body is busy doing, talk with a trusted family member or friend, someone who can listen to your worries and encourage positive thoughts about how your growing body benefits both you and baby.

What about Food for Baby?

As you choose healthy food to nourish your body, your body is busy preparing the perfect food to nourish your baby after birth. Nature's plan for the nourishment and nurturing of your baby is breastfeeding. Only in the last century have babies who were not breastfed had any chance of living. And only in the last fifty years has research examined breastfeeding and breast milk in comparison to artificial infant formula. The differences are astounding. The value and importance of breastfeeding for babies and for mothers is so well documented that we no longer talk of the *benefits of breastfeeding* but rather the *risks of not breastfeeding.*[5] (To read more, see Appendix D.)

Breast milk is the perfect food for babies. No artificial infant formula comes close. Breast milk contains every nutrient your baby needs, in just the right amount. For example, breast milk contains many essential fatty acids not present in any formula. Since fat is essential for brain development, it's no surprise that a number of well-designed research studies have documented higher IQs in breastfed babies. Breast milk is also rich with antibodies and macrophages that destroy bacteria and protect the baby. So it's no surprise either that formula-fed babies are at greater risk for respiratory infections, diarrhea, ear infections, and sudden infant death syndrome (SIDS). Formula-fed babies also have a greater risk of developing allergies, juvenile diabetes, and childhood cancers later in life.

And breast milk changes to match your baby's needs. Colostrum is extremely rich in antibodies and nutrients—perfect food for a newborn's tiny stomach, which is only the size of a walnut. Mothers of premature babies produce milk that's higher in fat than mothers of full-term babies. As breastfeeding is established, milk is higher in fat at the end of a feed and during the night. As baby gets older, the composition of milk is different than it was when baby was a newborn.

Breastfeeding makes a difference for mothers, too. Breastfeeding helps contract the uterus and reduce postpartum bleeding. Women who breastfeed their babies are at less risk of developing breast cancer and osteoporosis later in life (and the longer you breastfeed and the more babies you breastfeed, the better). Not only does breastfeeding provide health benefits, but most breastfeeding mothers describe how enjoyable it is as well. Every time you sit down to nurse your baby, oxytocin and prolactin are released. You feel relaxed, even a bit sleepy, ready to settle down and enjoy being with your baby.

If baby is breastfed exclusively—no formula or water between breastfeeding—and around the clock, levels of prolactin stay high enough to decrease the mother's fertility. Once baby starts on other food and starts sleeping through the night, fertility gradually returns. As a result, in parts of the world where women breastfeed exclusively and have no other form of birth control, babies usually come every two to three years.

Breastfeeding is simply and beautifully designed. You don't need to do anything to prepare your body for breast-feeding. There is no need to toughen nipples. Breasts and nipples come in all sizes and many shapes, and they all work beautifully. Nipples that don't stick out usually do so once baby latches on and begins to suck. Your baby comes fully equipped to nurse. Your baby will nuzzle and snuggle, find your nipple, open wide, and self-attach. Your baby knows just what to do.

That said, if women in your family or your friends haven't breastfed, you may want to take this time now to seek out and spend some time with women who are breastfeeding. (You might also purchase a book about breastfeeding. See Recommended Resources at the back of the book.) Seeing breastfeeding in action and hearing how breastfeeding fits into women's busy lives is invaluable. You'll probably hear that many women let most of the "dos and don'ts" of breastfeeding go in one ear and out the other. There are no rules. Eat and drink what you like. Breastfeeding has been part of women's everyday lives since the beginning of time, so you'll see that it surely isn't meant to turn your life upside down. It's nature's perfect plan for the nourishment and nurturing of your baby.

TESTING, TESTING, ONE, TWO, THREE

By the time you've reached these middle months of pregnancy, you've most likely chosen a caregiver, a birth site, and whom you'd like to be with you during labor and birth. The issue of prenatal appointments and tests comes into play in the middle months. The number of prenatal appointments and the range of tests you will face vary greatly with your choice of caregiver and birth site. If you chose an obstetrician and a hospital birth, you may find yourself making many more appointments for exams and tests than if you chose a midwife and a home birth or a birth center birth.

That said, all prenatal care will involve testing of some kind. The important thing is to know what's being done and why—and that you have the right to refuse any of it. Many tests were originally created for diagnosing problems in high-risk pregnancies. But with the increased medicalization of pregnancy, these tests have become routine for all pregnancies—high-risk or otherwise. This does not mean that the tests are risk-free. On the contrary: Some of them have not been thoroughly tested for safety, and some of them actually present risks to mother and baby. The American Academy of Pediatrics (AAP) is an organization of pediatricians and researchers who help improve health and safety for infants as well as children, adolescents, and young adults. When it comes to routine diagnostic prenatal testing, the AAP admits that "no test is perfect. There may be a problem even if the test does not show it. Also, a problem may not exist even if the test does show it."[6] This often presents an emotional risk. Because some tests can be unreliable, their unclear or misleading results can either decrease your confidence or give you a false assurance.

The Facts about Common Prenatal Tests

You have the right to know the details of how and why prenatal tests will be done and all the risks associated with each test. Following are some facts about tests you are likely to encounter.

Blood Tests

Blood tests check for a number of things, such as blood type (including whether you are Rh negative or positive) and iron levels that might need boosting. Some tests will determine the presence of sexually transmitted diseases or an infection. These tests are considered standard and helpful.

Urine Tests

A urine test (collecting a fresh urine sample and checking it for levels of sugar and protein) is done at each prenatal visit. High sugar levels in a pregnant woman's urine may indicate gestational diabetes. (See the bullet on glucose tolerance tests on page 78 for more details.) Most importantly, the urine test may also show the presence of protein. Especially in the last trimester, this can be a sign of preeclampsia (sometimes called pre-toxemia or pregnancy-induced hypertension). This is a serious disease, but it's rare and can be controlled if diagnosed. Because of this, the simple urine test is important.

Blood Pressure Checks

Blood pressure checks, along with urine tests, are considered essential components of prenatal care. High blood pressure may be related to stress or any number of other things, but in pregnancy, especially in the last trimester, it can mean preeclampsia. Controlling high blood pressure with bed rest and medication is sometimes necessary to keep it from developing into full-blown eclampsia, a very serious complication for mother and baby.

Cervical Checks

Cervical checks are seldom questioned by the women who go into a clinic or doctor's office, slip off their clothes, and don an exam gown every few weeks and then every week as they get closer to the birth. But these routine examinations are invasive and provide little useful information on their own in early pregnancy. Pregnancy is a time to protect your body from intrusion. Once in labor, your caregiver may check your cervix for dilation, but even then, measuring dilation doesn't determine how labor will progress or how long it will last.

Ultrasound Examinations (Sonograms)

Ultrasounds use sound waves produced by a moving a transducer across the mother's abdomen to create a picture of the baby inside the womb. These are often routine and popular tests, but it's important to weigh the pros and cons before you choose to have one done.

Both the World Health Organization and the National Institutes of Health agree that routine ultrasound testing has not been sufficiently evaluated to let the practice go unquestioned. For one, caregivers strongly disagree about the effect of ultrasound waves on fetal brains. A recent statement from the Federal Drug Administration (FDA) says, "Ultrasound is a form of energy, and even at low levels, laboratory studies have shown it can produce physical effects in the tissue, such as jarring vibrations and a rise in temperature." Because of this, the FDA declares that "prenatal ultrasounds can't be considered completely innocuous."[7] Also, some small studies in Europe and the United States have shown that ultrasound may cause developmental problems, such as delayed speech, as babies grow. *The Cochrane Library* does not recommend routine use of ultrasound in pregnancy, noting that while there are clear benefits to the judicious use of ultrasound, and there is no sound evidence that ultrasound is harmful in pregnancy, theoretical concern about potential hazards remains.[8]

On a more human note, expectant mothers approach ultrasound with different expectations and different emotions. It's wise to examine for your own feelings and motives before you make your decision. Some mothers choose to have ultrasounds because they're eager to "see" their babies and hear their heartbeats. It can be a tangible yet magical step toward building confidence and attachment, and they look forward to having photos of their babies in utero. Other mothers are much more hesitant, viewing ultrasound as an invasion of their babies' privacy and a "sciencing" of the intimate knowledge and ownership of pregnancy. They feel it's one more aspect of medicalization that lowers confidence in the natural ability of women's bodies to do the work of pregnancy and birth.

If you do wish to obtain an ultrasound photo of the baby, talk to your caregiver. Be leery of the new crop of unregulated, commercial sonogram shops. These "fun ultrasound" shops lure parents with the opportunity to "meet their baby" and the promise of "baby's first picture" as "a nice addition to any family album." Birth activist Marsden Wagner sounds the safety alarm: "At present, there is no known training or certification for users of ultrasound apparatus in any country. In other words, the birth machine has no license test for its drivers."[9]

Another aspect of ultrasound testing that meets mixed reactions is the opportunity to learn the baby's sex. Some mothers look forward to this important discovery, seeing it as a chance to know more about the babies growing inside them. They appreciate learning the sex early in the process, rather than in the emotional moments after the hard work of labor and birth. Some mothers value having the extra time to digest the information before their babies arrive. In contrast, other mothers want to preserve this surprise at all costs. They consider learning their babies' sex a beautiful reward after labor and birth. To them, finding out the sex is, again, an invasion of the special privacy of pregnancy. However you feel about this issue, know that using ultrasound to learn your baby's sex is an imperfect science, just like using ultrasound to calculate due dates and diagnose problems. For example, many parents have been told during ultrasounds that their babies are girls, only to be surprised to be holding boys in the moments after birth. As with all aspects of prenatal testing, think about what you'll do with the information if you choose to learn your baby's sex. And if you choose to have an ultrasound but not learn your baby's sex, make your wishes known to your caregiver so no one will unwittingly spoil the surprise during the procedure.

As you consider ultrasound testing and all its aspects, do it with the knowledge that it's an option—not a *requirement*—and that you have the right to refuse it. Since much of the information provided by ultrasounds does not ensure a baby's health and safety and is often subjectively evaluated, why routinely subject baby and mother to a procedure that has not been proven to be risk-free? Many women have stated that when they questioned or refused ultrasound testing, their caregivers made them feel guilty. These women were led to believe that choosing *not* to have the procedure done might endanger their babies. Heather shared her reaction after having an ultrasound: "I was surprised to find myself crying, and these were not tears of happiness," she recalled. "I felt like I'd given in on having the procedure done, not really believing it was necessary or right." If you feel undue pressure from a caregiver to have an ultrasound, consider seeking care elsewhere.

Multiple Marker Tests

Multiple marker tests (also known as maternal serum screening) look for the presence of proteins or hormones in the mother's blood that may signal a developmental problem. These tests have a high rate of false positives (results indicating there's something wrong when there isn't), which are discovered when further testing yields different results or when babies are born healthy despite the emotional toll the incorrect results placed on the mother. Before allowing this blood test to be done, you should think about what you would do with the information. You have a right to refuse this test. And if you have a positive result, you have the right to refuse further testing.

Amniocentesis

Amniocentesis is a procedure in which a small amount of fluid and cells are collected from the amniotic sac surrounding the fetus. Some caregivers warn women, especially those over the arbitrary age of thirty-five, that by not having an amniocentesis done, they are "at risk" of not finding out whether their babies have Down syndrome or other birth defects. What they may not emphasize is that this invasive test puts a woman's body and baby at risk of infection, bleeding, amniotic fluid leakage, fetal distress, and miscarriage. Because of these risks, it is *most* important to think about what you will do with the information before you agree to the procedure.

Glucose Tolerance Test

The glucose tolerance test screens for gestational diabetes. The mother drinks a special sugar mixture, and the level of glucose in her blood is measured. Many Canadian doctors have stopped using this test because research has not shown it to be necessary. Because women are overdiagnosed with gestational diabetes (at least 25 percent of pregnant women are treated for it in the U.S.) and because there's no evidence that taking preventive measures against gestational diabetes is beneficial ("untreated" women with high blood sugar have somewhat larger babies but no increased risk of cesarean or difficult labor), "it's probably not a good idea to be doing it routinely," says University of Washington family doctor Alfred Berg, who headed a government task force questioning the benefits of some prenatal testing.[10] *A Guide to Effective Care in Pregnancy and Childbirth* has this to say: "The available data provide no evidence to support the wide recommendation that all pregnant women should be screened for 'gestational diabetes' let alone that they be treated with insulin."[11]

The Danger of "Spoiling" Your Pregnancy

Sociologist Barbara Katz Rothman, who has studied the enviable Dutch system of birth, states that some Dutch midwives use the phrase "spoiling the pregnancy" when grappling with the issue of routine prenatal testing. They feel testing—especially misleading tests with false positives—robs the mother of joy, peace, and a relaxed relationship with the baby she's carrying inside.[12] One midwife Rothman interviewed said that after a baby is born, there will always be concerns throughout life—threats of accidents or illness and so on. The midwife mused, "It is a process, all life long, isn't it? Somehow or somewhere you have to let it go, you cannot control everything, and maybe you have to start to let it go at the beginning."

Rothman writes, "Americans cannot see the costs of ruining a pregnancy, of taking out a piece of the joy."[13] But many women *are* making the choice to trust in their pregnancies and decline some of the prenatal tests recommended to them. It's important to know that the tests presented to you as being "absolutely necessary" in one country may not be so in another country where the benefits and disadvantages have been better weighed. Also know that if an obstetrician believes a test is absolutely necessary, it may not be what a midwife believes. And it may not be what *you* believe.

RIPENING AND READYING: THE FINAL MONTHS

For some, the final months are the longest days of pregnancy. As your body grows into a ripened fruit, with your abdomen stretching to accommodate a growing baby inside you, you may feel beautiful but uncomfortable. Along with your hearty appetite, you may have indigestion from the pressure against your stomach. Pressure against your bladder and increased beverage consumption, which ensures healthy fluid exchange for the baby, bring frequent urination. Increased pressure in your abdomen and decreased blood return from your extremities may produce swelling in your ankles and feet. Backaches may be more frequent in response to the heaviness and positioning of the baby. Some women complain of leg cramps during times of rest, which may be caused by challenged calcium levels in their bodies.

For many mothers, the tiredness they felt during early pregnancy returns. The baby requires more and more of your assistance to run his or her body systems, and your energy wanes from carting around a little human being at every moment. The need for short periods of rest to let your body catch up with itself is just as important as the need for gentle exercise. Elevating your feet and propping up with pillows while lying on your left side will provide good support and blood flow for you and baby. (Lying on your left side takes the uterus's pressure off the main vein that passes through your body.)

Once the baby settles head-down in your uterus in the weeks before birth, you will notice less pressure on your lungs and stomach. You'll no longer feel a shortness of breath, but you'll feel a need to urinate more often. Your hormones are busy at work, helping your breasts produce colostrum in preparation for breastfeeding. The tissues in your pelvis are ripening and softening to prepare the birth canal for the baby's passage. The amniotic sac (also called the membrane or bag of waters) that surrounds the baby with protective fluid is busy exchanging its contents every six hours.

To help baby settle into the best position for labor—an occiput anterior position with the baby's face against your back and head against your belly—spend most of your time sitting upright and leaning a bit forward in the last weeks of pregnancy. Avoid semi-reclining, such as when you're lying on the sofa watching TV, slouched in the bucket seat of your car, or propped up in bed reading. A semi-reclined position makes it easy for baby to slide around into a posterior position, which in turn makes labor more difficult. So try to sit upright, supported by pillows when watching TV or traveling by car, and sleep on your side rather than propped on your back.

In the last weeks, you may begin to notice your uterus tightening. These are called Braxton-Hicks contractions. Your uterus has been tightening and releasing throughout pregnancy, but now it's noticeable. You are most likely to notice the tightening when you sit and relax or when you're moving quickly during the day. You also may notice an increase in vaginal discharge as your due date approaches. These signs all are part of nature's plan for the last weeks of pregnancy. (Note: Lots of contractions, a low backache, and an increase in vaginal discharge well before the last weeks of your pregnancy could mean preterm labor, and you should see your caregiver.)

The baby, who enjoyed a dance inside you in the earlier months, will continue some of those entertaining and athletic movements, but he or she may have quieter times as the birth draws closer and there's less and less space to explore. The baby will continue to grow toward the birth weight (a half-pound a week), and the heart, lung, and digestive systems will grow more and more able to independently function. The senses can already respond to light and sound and touch, and the sucking reflex matures as baby rehearses for the first meal at mama's breasts, which are busy readying milk that's full of nutrients and antibodies.

These final months are a time to pay loving attention to the work at hand of birthing your baby. Pregnancy should not be on the "back burner" of your life. If your maternity leave is limited and you're feeling well, you may choose to work until labor starts. Or you might choose to step back from work to center your mind and body, to rest and gather the energy for the birth ahead, and to "nest"—quietly attend to the final details of preparing your heart and home for this new family member. Throughout pregnancy, you've had to accommodate the changing shape of your body; now it's time to accommodate the changing shape of your life in general: How might the hours of your days (and nights) change in the months and years ahead? What are reasonable expectations about your home and appearance? What might lie ahead in relationships with your partner, your friends, and your extended family as you learn to accept and seek help in settling into your new role? What can you learn from this baby about yourself, your values, and your lifestyle? Now's the time to refigure what's most important.

What about Lovemaking These Days?

There was a time when pregnant women were told that intercourse in the last months might cause membrane rupture (breaking the bag of waters) and preterm labor. But there's no evidence that lovemaking in the last three months of pregnancy causes a difference in the length of pregnancy or the baby's birth weight or health.

This is good news for couples during this intense time in a relationship. Many couples feel the need to share physical affection in the final months of pregnancy, and having sex may lead to new ways of pleasuring each other and discovering each other's sexuality. It's an important time to affirm your love for each other, especially in a modern culture where thinness can be a commodity. The shape of a your fully pregnant body might make you feel unattractive, and your partner may fear that lovemaking will be awkward or that it might harm the baby, but there is nothing like sensitive and caring lovemaking to keep intimate lines of communication open. Use good sense in intimacy to find what works and feels best.

LAYING OUT CLOTHES
FOR THE BIG DANCE

Some women buy, borrow, and collect everything they think they'll need for the baby's room and wardrobe long before the third trimester. Other women prefer to wait until they are closer to the baby's arrival, be it a matter of energy levels, cultural preferences, or superstition. Likewise, some women will gather a roomful of brand-new items for their brand-new baby—T-shirts, onesies, sleepers, sweaters, hats, blankets, outfits, cloth or disposable diapers. Others will gladly receive

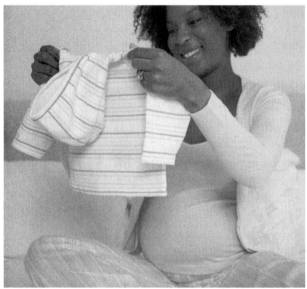

used items from friends, family, yard sales, and secondhand stores. A lot depends on habit, value systems, and income levels. But no matter when and how you assemble your baby's layette, laundering, folding, and arranging a newborn's clothes is good therapy for the last weeks of pregnancy.

Don't forget to collect a few items for yourself. These are the last days of maternity clothes—for better or worse. Your new body and new role after birth will no doubt require special clothes. One young mother shared her delight when her older sister bought her a stack of roomy, white cotton T-shirts, something she appreciated herself when nursing her own newborn. A clean T-shirt is relaxing, soft, and breathable; it goes with just about anything; and it makes things easily accessible during those first weeks of breastfeeding. "My sister looked back fondly on those first summer days with her little baby, when she'd shower and slip on one of those shirts and plop down to nurse, relaxed and refreshed," she shared.

AN ALTERNATIVE TO BABY SHOWERS

Our modern world can be so fast-paced that we forget to take thoughtful time to celebrate and honor important life transitions, such as the one you face during these last days of pregnancy. The modern baby shower came into vogue after World War II, possibly in response to the baby boom of that era, but there's evidence that ancient Egyptians and Romans practiced gift-giving to newborns.

Although baby showers allow friends and family to share in the joy of welcoming a new life, they—like so many of our modern celebrations—often fail to really address the importance of the event they celebrate. These gatherings should be times of inspiration, encouragement, and strengthening for a mother-to-be, but they seem to have become marketable events that the baby-goods industry has capitalized on.

We need to take the time to do a more ritual honoring of a pregnant woman and the work she's doing and is about to do. Kathryn Hall of the Birth Project (see page 23) tells of a naming ceremony celebrated with parents of newborns, but it's an event you could modify and incorporate into a baby shower during the last months of pregnancy. "I learned of the naming ceremony from a woman from Ghana, but it's used all over the world in different ways. It calls people together to educate, to inspire, and to support them when they're getting ready to do something different, something new. And having a baby is something new!" says Hall.[14] Rather than just eating, unwrapping gifts, and playing games like usual, adding elements of the naming ceremony lends some symbolic importance to your gathering.

A naming ceremony gathers (or creates) a mother's support group—people who will support you and your child during the life journey that lies ahead. Hall suggests the group form a circle and help pass around items that have special meaning about the future with your baby:

- A little bowl of cinnamon for you to taste from, symbolizing the bitter things you won't like, the difficulties you'll encounter;
- A little bowl of sugar, symbolizing the things you'll love about being a mother;

- A little bowl of salt, symbolizing individuality—the way you'll use your unique judgment;
- A little bowl of honey, symbolizing the richness and the hard but rewarding work that lies ahead; and
- A bowl of water to drink from, symbolizing the things over which you'll have no control in the years ahead.

After the tasting comes an important part of the ceremony—the empty crystal bowl. Hall explains that the empty bowl symbolizes that when we come into the world, we are empty. "And as you go through life, things will eventually come into your bowl and *that* will be who you are." The bowl is passed around, and each person places a symbolic stone into it, perhaps sharing a word of encouragement or support to the mother. When the Birth Project's "Sister Friends" step into a relationship with a pregnant woman, they place into the bowl small stones that symbolize prayer—the prayers they commit to offer for this new life. This becomes a powerful statement affirming that this baby truly belongs to a community, that this mother does not have to care for the baby all by herself, and that others stand beside her with their love and prayers.

Candles are also symbolic items in the Birth Project community, and you can adapt their special candle ritual for your own event as well. "Prior to the birth of the baby, special candles are given to a group of people who are going to pray for the baby while it's being born," says Hall. "So a mother would identify five to ten people who will have this special role in her life. She gives them the birth candle, and at the point when she goes into active labor, someone will be instructed to call the rest of the folks who have a candle. They'll light it and keep it going until they hear that the baby has arrived here safely." These people then save their candle-holders and give them to the child when he or she is older, perhaps at a birthday celebration or a difficult time. This symbol lets the child know that he or she was valued and thought of right from the beginning. So, you may wish to be a gift-giver at your own shower, placing candles into your shower attendees' hands with a request that they light them when your labor begins.

CAN YOU HEAR THE MUSIC?

These final weeks before birth are like a preparation for a big dance. The dance floor is ready—the past nine months of eating well, exercising, and resting have been a time for preparation. The musicians are practiced and gathered—mother and baby have been warming up for months, learning how to make the best music together. And at just the right time, when things are completely ready, the dance of labor and birth will begin, and the players who have been rehearsing for all these weeks will delight in seeing each other's faces. For now, enjoy the last days before the dance, and take heart in the confidence that you are ready and able to do this very good work of normal, natural birth.

Chapter 6

PREPARING FOR LABOR AND BIRTH

That is what learning is.
You suddenly understand something
you've understood all your life,
but in a new way.
–Doris Lessing

You may not realize it yet, but you've been preparing for the work of labor and birth throughout your pregnancy—in fact, throughout your life. The power and wisdom you need to give birth is already in you. But like most women, you may need to do some thinking, talking, reading, and more thinking to find and use these inner resources.

Everyday life is excellent training for childbirth. Chances are you've done plenty of simple (and not-so-simple) hard work over the years. Every challenge you face and every demand you meet prepares you for the work of birth and mothering. You'll draw on all that you are as you help your baby out of your belly and into your arms. And you may well find that this work transforms you into a stronger, more capable, more confident woman.

LISTEN TO YOUR BODY

Throughout your pregnancy you react to what you feel physically and emotionally. You move differently in response to your changing size and shape. You eat differently in response to nausea, sensitivity to smells, and changing tastes. You sleep differently in response to increasing fatigue or discomfort. You pat, stroke, and talk to your belly when you feel your baby squirm and kick. Your body tells you what to do and when to do it, and you are free to listen and follow your body's lead.

In the same way, your body will lead you into and guide you through labor and birth. During the last months of your pregnancy, a precisely choreographed dance takes place inside you. Your hormones shift, your uterus begins to contract, and your cervix softens. Your baby stores fat and his or her lungs mature. As your baby begins to outgrow your womb, he or she turns head-down and drops lower in your pelvis. Your baby's getting ready to leave the warm protection of your womb, and you're getting ready to care for your baby in a new way.

LISTEN TO OTHER WOMEN

While on a basic level, all you really need to do is listen to your body and follow its lead, giving birth isn't meant to be taken for granted. You'll naturally have questions as you approach birth. You may wonder, "How will I know I'm in labor? What will it feel like? What should I do?"

Getting answers to these questions can help you learn what to expect, tune in to your body, and build confidence in your ability to do the work your body's designed for. In the past women learned the details of labor and birth from their own mothers and from women who had become wise about birth from years of childbearing and attending to birthing women.

Judith's Story of Learning about Birth

In 1917 my grandmother Nora, who was expecting her first child, asked her mother, Nellie, about birth. And my great-grandmother Nellie shared her five birth stories with Nora. Over time, surrounded by the quiet comfort and encouragement of her mother and sisters, Nora birthed six children in the bed where they were conceived.

By the time Nora's daughter Ruth, my mother, grew into a woman, babies were brought into the world differently. My mother gave birth to her own six children in a hospital, alone except for the medical staff who told her what to do and who were, in reality, strangers. Nora, having had her babies naturally and at home, had little advice to offer my mother. She knew nothing about "modern" hospital birth. Although my mother, like Nora, labored without medication, she was anesthetized for all six births because that was standard hospital procedure.

The birth culture of my mother's childbearing years disconnected her from the birth wisdom of her own family. The lost stories included not just Nora's and Nellie's, but also my mother's own story. My mother never shared her birth stories with me or my sisters. Robbed of consciousness, joy, and the ability to remember her births, she felt she had nothing to share.

I grew up to be a nurse. Despite my nursing training, I learned my most important lesson about birth when I attended one—just one—woman who gave birth without medication and with her husband at her side. It was 1966, and I was a nursing student. From that day on I carried with me the life-changing image of a strong woman laboring and birthing naturally.

When I became pregnant and wanted more information about the experience of pregnancy and childbirth, I signed up for a Lamaze class. My nursing classes had taught me the facts of anatomy and physiology. And my Lamaze classes went on to teach me about the stages of labor and how to deal with the pain of contractions. But that one woman birthing naturally in 1966 taught me my most valuable lesson: the lesson of confidence in my body and in my innate ability to give birth.

After considering all that I'd learned, I chose to give birth naturally. And like my great-grandmother Nellie, I shared my birth stories with my daughters. I believe that sharing my confidence and my knowledge of women's ability to give birth naturally is among the most important things I have given them. My daughters have learned about birth in simple faith, by listening to birth stories and being surrounded their whole lives by women and men who trust birth.

When my eldest daughter, Mary, became pregnant, she asked me the same questions my grandmother Nora had asked my great-grandmother Nellie in 1917. Like Nora, Mary got her questions answered. And I, like many generations of mothers before me, stood beside my daughter during her pregnancy, labor, and birth to offer encouragement, comfort, and support. Though we couldn't restore our family's lost stories, we did restore our family's tradition of women helping women on the road to motherhood. Our broken link in the circle of birthing women was repaired.

With confidence in her abilities and help from her family, Mary gave birth to a daughter and blessed her with the ancestral name of Nora. In time she had three more daughters: Molly, Maggie, and Cate. (For Mary's first three birth stories, see pages 57 and 60.)

Mary now shares her story again and again with her sisters, her friends, and you. And Mary has already shared her birth wisdom with her little daughters. When Cate was born, six-year-old Nora sat at her mother's side and welcomed her sister into the world. Molly and Maggie, wide-eyed and joyful, helped dry Cate and place her in their mother's arms.

Learning from Women You Know

If you want to give birth naturally, and you know women who've experienced normal birth, they will be your most important teachers. Talk with them. Ask the women in your family about their births. If your family has lived in the United States for a while, you may have to go back a few generations to written birth records or handed-down family stories. If your parents or grandparents grew up in other countries, you may be fortunate enough to hear family stories of natural birth firsthand. In such stories, there's a wealth of knowledge to be uncovered and reclaimed.

And what about stories from women who've experienced medical birth? Listen to these, too; you'll learn a lot from them. But don't let them frighten you; remember that the women telling these stories probably see birth through a different lens than you do. Note how these stories differ from the stories of women who have given birth normally.

As you listen to and learn from women who've gone before you, think about whether their strengths and hopes resemble yours. You may be surprised at what emerges— ways you'd like to emulate, ways you'd like to do things differently, ways you can make positive progress in your journey toward birth.

CONSIDER CHILDBIRTH EDUCATION

Chances are you're wondering how childbirth education fits into the scheme of preparing for normal birth. Formal childbirth education sprang up to fill the void created when several decades of birth stories were lost. During the first half of the twentieth century, most women were heavily medicated for labor and anesthetized for birth, and they simply had little—if any—memory or practical information about childbirth to share.

When Lamaze and other childbirth classes were first offered in the early 1960s, they gave women basic information about birth physiology and coping strategies, like breathing and relaxing, to enable them to labor and give birth without medication. Husbands attended classes, too, and learned to "coach" their wives through contractions and provide emotional support throughout labor.

The information was basic, and the skills were simple. In the 1960s and 1970s, that was all women needed to help them give birth confidently.

But times have changed. Though some harmful and/or useless medical birth practices have fallen by the wayside since 1960, new ones have appeared to take their place. The technology that has grown up around U.S. birth during the past fifty years has made it progressively harder to give birth normally. Though a growing body of research supports natural birth and a growing number of women are learning about, experiencing, and sharing stories about normal birth, many *more* women continue to hand over their births to obstetricians and hospitals.

Today, childbirth education needs to provide more than basic knowledge and skills. Today, the most valuable childbirth classes will also help women understand the possible negative influence of technology on their ability to give birth normally and equip them with strategies to minimize unnecessary interventions.

Should You Attend Childbirth Classes?

Ideally, women shouldn't have to take formal classes to give birth confidently. But we aren't living in an ideal world. In a culture that relies on technology in both health and illness, childbirth classes can do much to help you recognize your own abilities and trust your own wisdom.

Our great-grandmothers, surrounded by the birth wisdom of women who'd gone before them, didn't need childbirth classes. But they also didn't face the cultural challenges birthing women face today. Should you attend childbirth classes? We recommend that you ask yourself the following questions to help you decide.

- Did you grow up believing that your body works beautifully? That its functions are normal, natural, and healthy in general—and in particular regarding childbirth?
- Do you know and trust women who have given birth naturally and confidently?
- Have you talked with a woman who had a baby with a midwife's help?
- Do you know other people who believe in the normalcy of birth and in women's ability to birth naturally?
- Will your birth site allow you freedom to respond to your body's signals however you need to as you move through labor?
- Will you be supported during birth by family and/or friends who are confident and knowledgeable, like you?

If you've answered yes to all these questions, then you might not need formal childbirth education. If not, classes may help you.

What to Look for in an Educator

If you want to give birth naturally, you should look for a childbirth educator who's both knowledgeable about and committed to normal birth. She should believe, with you, that you can do the work of labor and birth without medical intervention. She should respect your ability to make decisions that are right for you. She should be an advocate who shares *all* the information you need to make truly informed decisions.

How do you know if your teacher has knowledge and skill in normal birth? Many childbirth educators are nurses, but not all good teachers are nurses—and not all nurses are good teachers. There are many organizations that train childbirth educators, but Lamaze International offers the only certification program for childbirth educators that's accredited by the National Commission for Certifying Agencies (NCCA). Accreditation by NCCA is assurance that the Lamaze childbirth educator certification program meets the highest possible standards for assessing professional competence. If your teacher is a Lamaze Certified Childbirth Educator (LCCE), she has demonstrated her competence by passing a rigorous examination. She has proven her ability to:

- promote childbearing as a normal, natural, healthy process that profoundly affects women and their families;
- help women and families discover and use strategies that facilitate normal, natural, healthy pregnancy, birth, breastfeeding, and early parenting;
- help women and families understand how interventions and complications influence the normal course of pregnancy, birth, breastfeeding, and early parenting;
- give information and support that encourage attachment between babies and their families;
- help women and their families make informed birth decisions;
- advocate for women and families who want normal, natural, healthy, fulfilling childbirth;
- design, teach, and evaluate a course in Lamaze preparation that increases women's confidence and ability to give birth.

There are, of course, other excellent teachers who are not Lamaze certified. What's most important is that your educator trusts birth, is a good teacher, and has confidence in you. With those qualities will come the inspiration and motivation you need to help you prepare for the birth of your baby.

What to Look for in a Class

Like a favorite class you had growing up, on a subject you loved with a teacher you admired, the right childbirth class should make you smile, relax, and embrace what you're learning. It's not a place for lectures or tests. Rather, it's a place for discovery, questions, discussion, and confident anticipation. The best classes needn't provide vast amounts of technical information, but they should help you untangle the web of modern obstetrics and figure out what's best for you. You should leave your class assured rather than fearful.

What should you learn in a childbirth class? We believe that overall, childbirth classes should provide knowledge and skills that build your confidence in your ability to give birth. The most important thing you should learn is the simple story of normal birth. You should discuss the care practices that support normal birth as well as strategies to keep birth as normal as possible even if difficulties arise. You should learn and practice ways to find comfort during labor. Classes should also include basic breastfeeding information and tips on communicating with caregivers. A good childbirth class gives women all the information they need to make truly informed decisions. Finally, good classes are small (preferably no more than ten couples) and interactive.

We recommend that you avoid taking a class that undermines your confidence in any way. Be wary of classes that focus on hospital protocols, possible complications, and medical interventions; learning about labor and childbirth shouldn't focus on what might go wrong. Be wary of a teacher who's quick to remind the class that the doctor and hospital always know what's best for you; only *you* know what's best for you, and medical practices aren't always based on best evidence. Be wary of large class sizes, which are likely to prevent your questions and concerns from being addressed adequately. Be wary of classes that suggest that birth is safe only in a hospital, that routine interventions are necessary for a safe birth, that epidurals do not affect babies, or that pain plays no role in normal birth; these claims simply aren't true.

If you're considering attending a "Lamaze" class in your area, make sure it's genuine Lamaze. A real Lamaze course is taught by a Lamaze Certified Childbirth Educator and is based on the Lamaze Philosophy of Birth (see page vii). A hallmark of Lamaze classes is commitment to presenting evidence-based information. Lamaze classes prepare women for normal birth, help women understand the influence of obstetric practices on the natural,

Be especially cautious if you are considering attending classes at a hospital. Many hospital classes are simply too large, and hospital administrators often pressure teachers to prepare women for the birth experience in that particular hospital. As a result, teachers must often withhold evidence and options. For instance, if a hospital's policy is continuous electronic fetal monitoring (EFM) for all women, its teachers are expected to discuss the importance of EFM for safety. And naturally, they're expected *not* to discuss the important evidence that continuous EFM doesn't benefit babies and increases maternal risks. The women who attend these classes never learn the full story.

normal process of birth, help women make informed decisions that are right for them, and help women navigate the maze of modern obstetrics. Be wary of "Lamaze" classes that spend a lot of time practicing relaxation and breathing and little or no time building your confidence or discussing how to promote, protect, and support normal birth.

Making Your Choice

As you choose a birth class, talk to a few women who've taken classes in different settings. Talk to a midwife or other caregiver. Talk with the childbirth educators themselves. Ask yourself how the class you're considering fits your values. And remember that if the class you choose turns out to be a poor fit, you can change classes.

The following chapters provide a quick snapshot of the information covered in a Lamaze course. Your own classes will provide a forum for discussion, for questioning, for strengthening your communication skills, for practicing comfort measures, and for building your confidence.

Chapter 7

THE SIMPLE STORY OF BIRTH

*When I crossed the finish line of my first marathon,
I felt exactly the same exhilaration I felt when Ben was
born. I did it! The feeling of accomplishment I experienced
after natural childbirth gave me strength and confidence
for years afterward, whenever I wasn't sure I was up to
a new challenge. The positive struggle of working with
your body in labor and birth can be a reward in itself.
And then add the joy of having a healthy baby!*
—Debby Amis

HERE'S WHAT HAPPENS

During the last weeks of pregnancy a series of physical
changes sets the stage for your baby's birth. The changes
happen slowly but predictably, and each change is a vitally
important event in the drama of labor and birth. Your baby
is ready to be born. And your body knows this. Together,
your body and your baby dance into motion.

Dramatic hormonal shifts orchestrate this entire process.
In the final weeks of pregnancy, your body begins to release
more prostaglandins to soften your cervix. Your baby settles
lower in your pelvis. This is very early labor, and nature has
designed it to happen gradually and deliberately. You may
notice strong (but typically not painful) uterine contractions.
Sometimes they become rhythmic, then go away. This is
exactly what your body needs to do.

You may not realize you're in labor at first. Women who
do recognize early labor contractions often describe them as
mild, cramplike pains that start deep in the abdomen and
move downward toward the groin. If the back of your baby's

head is facing your back (occiput posterior position), you may feel early contractions as back pain.

Labor—especially early labor—is a process that's easily affected by your surroundings. Most mammals seek quiet and privacy when they're in labor, and if they sense danger of any kind, labor stops. This frees them to move to safety, or lets them wait until danger passes to deliver their babies. Human labor fits this pattern: Early on, it can be shut down by anxiety, fear, or anything that makes you feel unsafe. That's why it's important to choose a birth site and caregiver that help you feel confident and secure.

As labor progresses, your body releases increasing amounts of oxytocin to make your uterus contract (tighten and relax) in a steady rhythm. As your body releases more and more oxytocin, your contractions grow stronger and stronger. These contractions slowly efface (thin) and dilate (open) your softened cervix and encourage your baby to inch downward in your pelvis.

Contractions are like waves at the beach. Early contractions are like gentle waves. Gradually, the contractions grow stronger and closer together—the waves grow higher and deeper and more difficult to ride. When your contractions are lasting a minute long and are less than five minutes apart (from the beginning of one contraction to the beginning of the next), and are gaining strength, you're in active labor. It can take anywhere from a few hours to a few days to reach this point in labor.

As oxytocin surges and your contractions grow more painful, the high oxytocin and pain levels signal your brain to release hormones called endorphins. Endorphins decrease pain perception, moderate oxytocin release (giving you and your uterus little breaks), and help you enter a dreamlike state. Endorphins help you turn inward, act more intuitively, and find a rhythm as you cope with contractions.

At exactly the right time, as your baby rotates and descends through your pelvis, you begin to feel an urge to push. Pushing is a reflex, and like other reflexive behaviors (such as sneezing), it doesn't need to be taught. It happens naturally and is, in fact, difficult to stop. Responding to this urge, you move and change position frequently to find the best position for pushing. If you follow your instincts, you're likely to give birth upright to take advantage of gravity, and you may squat or get into other positions that enlarge your pelvis.

It's common to feel anxious during the pushing stage. This sudden anxiety stimulates the release of catecholamines (stress hormones) in you and your baby. At this stage, unlike in early labor, stress hormones actually help the process. French obstetrician Michel Odent theorizes that a mammal far along in labor is very vulnerable to predators, so it's essential for mammals to deliver their young quickly.[1] A catecholamine surge helps hasten birth.

Catecholamines make you more alert, more focused, and extremely strong to help you push your baby out. Your baby emerges face-down, then rotates ninety degrees so his or her shoulders can deliver one at a time. The rest of your baby's body slides out quickly. This trip through the birth canal squeezes amniotic fluid out of your baby's lungs to make room for air. The cooler temperature outside your body, a slight decrease in oxygen from you, and high catecholamines cause your baby to take an instinctive first breath. Catecholamines also make your newborn baby very alert.

When your baby is placed on your abdomen, his or her weight helps your uterus contract to deliver your placenta. Your body heat keeps your baby warm. Skin-to-skin with you, your baby's breathing and heart rate stay more stable than they would if he or she were separated from you and placed in a warming bed. Your baby's head and hand movements stimulate your body to produce prolactin, which helps your breasts make milk, and to continue producing oxytocin, which keeps your uterus tight to prevent bleeding and also helps your milk let down. If your baby is left undisturbed, skin-to-skin with you, he or she will slowly and methodically crawl to your breast and latch on.[2]

High levels of all these hormones—endorphins, catecholamines, oxytocin, and prolactin—contribute to the euphoria you feel holding your baby right after birth. And high levels of endorphins in your breast milk ease your baby's transition to life outside your womb.

In this story of normal birth, labor unfolds quite naturally. No machines time or rate your progress. No experts tell you what to do or what not to do. No one takes your baby from you. It's an ancient story of a strong, confident woman and a competent baby who both know just what to do. It's all good news.

PAIN WITH A PURPOSE

What may *not* seem like good news is the pain woven throughout this story. Most pregnant women worry about the pain of labor and birth. No one enjoys pain, and people go to great lengths to avoid it. But make no mistake: Pain is a normal, healthy, and necessary part of childbirth. In fact, pain is *central* to the elegant design of birth; it's not an unfortunate side effect.

At the beginning of labor, pain lets you know that it's not just another day. Knowing you're in labor gives you time to gather the help you need and to go to a safe, secure place. Without pain to signal the start of labor, many more babies would be born in cars, shopping malls, and on the street.

Like other pain in your life, childbirth pain protects you. If you accidentally touch a hot stove, the pain makes you instinctively pull your hand away to prevent a burn. If you develop a blister on your foot, the pain makes you change the way you walk to protect your foot from further injury. If you're in labor, the pain of a contraction makes you move, rub, or moan in an effort to get comfortable. Your actions ease the pain a bit and help you get from one contraction to the next—even stronger—contraction.

Coping with pain gives your body the green light to increase oxytocin release, which causes stronger, more effective, and more painful contractions—and ultimately the release of endorphins, "nature's narcotic." At the same time, your movement helps your baby rotate and descend gradually and gently. Every time you move, the diameter of your pelvis changes, giving your baby a little room to wiggle through your birth canal.

Medicating the pain away disrupts labor. If you can't feel the pain of contractions or the pressure of your baby's descent, you can't respond to it. Your body doesn't know to release more oxytocin, and your birth canal is more vulnerable to damage. Removing labor pain also prevents endorphin release, depriving you of the natural high of childbirth. Remove the pain at any point in the journey, and you remove the signals your body needs to keep labor progressing and to protect itself and your baby.

Why should you face and feel labor pain? The answer is simple: Pain is a key element of nature's perfect plan for birth. Pain promotes the progress of labor, protects the birth canal and the baby from trauma, and ensures high levels of oxytocin and endorphins. Coping with labor pain naturally improves your odds for a faster and easier birth, an alert baby, a healthy you, and a successful start to breastfeeding.

TRUST: A TRUSTY TOOL

"Self-trust is the first secret of success...," writes Ralph Waldo Emerson. We agree. Trust in the natural process of birth and in your ability to give birth naturally is the best tool you have in your quest for a healthy, satisfying birth. In other words: Time is your friend in labor. Fear is not.

How long does normal labor last? Exactly as long as it needs to. There's wide variation in the length of normal labor. How your labor goes depends on many factors. The strength of your contractions and the size and position of your baby are two obvious ones. But other factors are equally important: security, confidence, freedom to move and find comfort however you like, emotional and physical support. All these things help labor progress.

British anthropologist Sheila Kitzinger believes that the most destructive technology used in birth is the clock.[3] Only in the Western world (particularly in the United States) is labor described in terms of time. For most of the world's women, clocks aren't central to birth. It takes time—sometimes lots of it—for your cervix to soften, for your hormones to rise, for your baby to maneuver, and for you to get into a laboring mind.[4] You can expect early labor to take longer and active labor to move more quickly. But outside these expectations, it makes sense to forget the clock and appreciate the time labor takes.

Remember that women have been doing this work forever. You have every reason to feel safe and confident. You are made for giving birth. Like countless generations of women before you, you will know what to do as your labor progresses. We encourage you to let go of worry and trust your body and soul. We bet you'll be glad you did.

Chapter 8

KEEPING BIRTH NORMAL

One cannot actively help a woman give birth.
The goal is to avoid disturbing her unnecessarily.
—Michel Odent

Today's typical American maternity care aims to help birthing women—but much of it actually disturbs them and makes labor more difficult and complicated. Research has clearly identified many care practices that are ineffective or harmful, as well as many that promote, protect, and support normal birth. We explain both in this chapter, with tips on how to avoid the former and achieve the latter.

The helpful care practices described on the following pages are simple and backed by strong evidence, but unfortunately, they're relatively uncommon in American obstetrics. We realize that these care practices may be unfamiliar to you and/or your caregiver, so we cite a great deal of research to support the claims we make. Our gold standard is the Cochrane Collaboration's *A Guide to Effective Care in Pregnancy and Childbirth*, which summarizes current maternity research findings and makes recommendations for practice. (See Appendix A.) You'll notice that we cite this resource—and many other respected sources—repeatedly.

Lamaze's six recommended care practices are a guide for creating a birth environment that lets you tap into your innate birth wisdom and give birth simply. Regardless of your baby's size, your labor's length and complexity, or your confidence level, these care practices will help you keep your labor and birth as normal as possible.

CARE PRACTICE 1: LABOR BEGINS ON ITS OWN

Letting your body go into labor spontaneously is almost always the best way to know that your baby is ready to be born and that your body is ready for labor. In the vast majority of pregnancies, labor will start only when all the players—your baby, your uterus, your hormones, and your placenta—are ready. Naturally, labor usually goes better and mother and baby usually end up healthier when all systems are go for birth.

Every Day Is Important

Every day of the last weeks of pregnancy is vital to your baby's and body's preparation for birth. During this time you pass antibodies to your baby to help him or her fight infections. Your baby gains weight and strength, stores iron, and his or her suck-and-swallow coordination matures. Your baby's lungs mature, too, and begin to produce a substance called surfactant, which helps the tiny alveoli (air sacs) stay inflated after birth.

Your maturing baby and aging placenta trigger a prostaglandin increase, which softens your cervix, and an estrogen increase and progesterone decrease, which make your uterus more sensitive to oxytocin. Your uterus contracts in response to the oxytocin, which makes your cervix efface (thin) and dilate (open). Your baby moves down into your pelvis.

New physical sensations at the end of pregnancy may make you feel antsy for birth. You may notice more vaginal secretions, colostrum leaking from your breasts, and interrupted sleep. After your baby drops, your clothes may fit differently, you may feel less short of breath, and you may have to urinate more often because your baby is crowding your bladder. You may also notice a burst of energy. This "nesting" urge is nature's way of helping you finish up baby preparations.

As labor approaches, you may notice some bloody show (blood-tinged vaginal discharge) or you may lose the mucous plug that sealed off the small opening of your cervix throughout pregnancy. Passing your mucous plug doesn't cause pain or discomfort, and it doesn't necessarily mean labor is about to start. You may also have diarrhea or very soft bowel movements; this is nature's way of making room in your pelvis.

Early Labor: Do Not Disturb

Many people believe that labor always begins with a woman's water breaking. Actually, only about one in six labors starts this way. (For most women the bag of water breaks sometime in active labor, and for some women it doesn't happen until the baby's head emerges.) If your water does break before contractions start, contractions will most likely start within twenty-four hours. When water breaks on its own, it's usually a small tear that only leaks during a contraction. So even if your water breaks early in labor, your amniotic sac continues to cushion your baby and your birth canal.

In early labor you're likely to feel contractions that are gentle and irregular, although they may become strong enough to stop you in your tracks and then fade. Such contractions may make you think you're in active labor, but chances are you're not. Active labor is marked by strong, regular contractions that do not fade, but rather grow stronger and closer together.

Early labor contractions can come and go for days or even weeks. Off-and-on contractions are sometimes called false labor, but really, there's nothing false about early labor. A long, sporadic early labor is normal, and it helps your body accomplish important preliminary work.

You may be quite unaware of your early labor, and it may go fairly quickly. Or you may find it long and tiring. Fatigue and frustration can make a long early labor difficult. It helps to alternate rest and activity to conserve your strength. It also helps to remember that this early stage is both important and normal.

Anthropologist Sheila Kitzinger recalls a midwife's story of early labor from a birth she attended: "We spent much of the first stage in the garden, putting in bedding plants together. Then we came in and made some cookies and cleaned up the kitchen. By that time, I could tell from her breathing that she was nearly fully dilated."[1]

It's very important not only to let your labor start on its own, but also to be undisturbed early in your labor. If you feel safe and secure and have some measure of privacy, your stress hormones stay low and your labor can progress unhindered.

When you're at home supported by family, friends, or a professional doula—people who understand and trust birth—you're more likely to feel safe and relaxed. Stay at home as long as you continue to feel safe and secure there. Here are some easy things you can do to help you through early labor:

- Eat and drink to keep up your energy.
- Alternate rest and activity.
- Remind yourself that your body knows what to do.

If you're not planning a home birth, remember that going to the hospital too soon starts a medical clock ticking and increases your risk of medical intervention. It's time to travel to your birth center or hospital when your contractions are close together, are growing and staying stronger, and are increasingly difficult to handle.

When Labor Is Induced

If your labor is induced (started artificially), it becomes a medical event and proceeds quite differently from spontaneous labor. There are valid health reasons for induction (see page 107), but most inductions today are elective (chosen for non-medical reasons).

Most inductions today are done for social reasons: Women are tired of being pregnant and eager to meet their babies, caregivers prefer to schedule births during the week and during the day, or women want to schedule births for convenient dates. Many women are told elective induction has no downside. This is not true.

Elective induction carries many risks and disadvantages. The important events of late pregnancy and early labor do not have a chance to unfold. Your cervix may not be sufficiently soft. Your uterus may not be highly sensitive to oxytocin. Your baby may not be mature enough. A baby who's even slightly early is more likely than a full-term baby to have problems adjusting to life outside the womb. Your baby may have trouble breastfeeding and is three times more likely to die in the first year of life than a full-term baby.[2]

Labor is usually induced with intravenous (IV) Pitocin, a synthetic oxytocin. Pitocin contractions feel stronger and peak more quickly than natural contractions. Also, your uterus never totally relaxes between contractions, which puts more stress on both your uterus and your baby. Pitocin doesn't cross the blood-brain barrier, so your brain doesn't get the message (as it would with natural oxytocin) to release endorphins. Without endorphins, you have no natural pain relief and thus have a greater need for pain medication. When your labor is induced, you also require IV fluids, continuous electronic fetal monitoring (EFM), and sometimes a bladder catheter. Finally, you'll likely be restricted to bed and prevented from actively working with your labor.

Labor induction alters not only the process of labor and birth, but also postpartum events. Pitocin short-circuits your natural hormone release, so neither you nor your baby experience the catecholamine surge necessary for energy and alertness after birth. Your baby is less likely to crawl to your breast and latch on and is less likely to make the hand and head movements on your chest that stimulate continued oxytocin release, which controls bleeding and helps your milk let down. This can complicate the start of breastfeeding.

There are, of course, some good reasons for inducing labor. The American College of Obstetricians and Gynecologists (ACOG) believes labor should be induced only when it's riskier for baby to stay in the uterus than to be born. This is true when the water breaks and labor doesn't begin, when pregnancy has reached forty-two weeks, when mother's blood pressure is high and can't be controlled by medication and bed rest, when mother has health problems (like diabetes) that can't be controlled and could harm her baby, when mother has a uterine infection, or when baby has a growth problem.[3] Suspecting a very large baby (macrosomia) is *not* a good reason for induction.[4] Research shows that inducing for "overdue" babies (before forty-two weeks) increases labor complications and cesareans without improving neonatal outcomes.[5]

Unless you or your baby has a health problem that necessitates induction, it makes sense to wait patiently for your labor to start on its own. Even if your due date has passed and you're longing to hold your baby, remember that nature has good reasons for the wait.

CARE PRACTICE 2: FREEDOM OF MOVEMENT THROUGHOUT LABOR

Why Movement Works

Moving in labor serves two very important purposes. First, it helps you cope with increasingly strong and painful contractions, which signals your body to keep labor going. Second, it helps gently wiggle your baby into your pelvis and through your birth canal.

When allowed to move freely, women instinctively respond to labor pains the same way we deal with pain in our daily lives: squirming to find a comfortable position in an uncomfortable chair, walking differently to protect a blistered toe, rocking to ease gas pains, rubbing to relieve a headache. Walking, changing position, squatting, rocking, rubbing, and swaying are effective ways to work with many kinds of pain, not just labor pain. Without freedom of movement, it's difficult to cope with ordinary pain—and nearly impossible to handle labor without medical interventions.

In labor, movement provides other benefits, too: Not only does it help you find comfort, it also hastens your baby's journey through your body in a way that protects both of you from injury. Regardless of your pelvis size or your baby's size, your baby must rotate to get through your pelvis. Your uterus contracts more efficiently[6] and your baby rotates and descends more effectively when you move than when you keep still during labor.

According to birth activist and midwife Mary Kroger, "Often instinctively a mother will assume a position that favors faster, more effective labor."[7] Without direction, a woman in labor will follow her body's lead to move among standing, sitting, crouching, squatting, and kneeling. And she'll move more as the birth of her baby approaches.[8]

There are no studies that directly compare the outcomes of labors with and without freedom of movement, but evidence does show that women find movement helpful. According to *A Guide to Effective Care in Pregnancy and Childbirth*, "freedom of movement and choice of positions in labor" is "likely to be beneficial,"[9] and one study reported that walking appeared to be safe and that 99 percent of the women who walked in labor liked it and would walk in a subsequent labor.[10] Unfortunately, the *Listening to Mothers* survey found that only 30 percent of women had freedom of movement in labor. The reason women gave most often for not moving in labor was "being hooked up to machines."[11] Imagine trying to navigate a dance floor tethered to an IV pole!

> "When my daughter Mary was in labor, she rapidly and rhythmically shook her arms and hands with each contraction—a movement she'd never done before. My great-aunt Esther chanted, 'Oh my God! Oh Mama!' as she walked around her dining room table. Rhythmic movement like rocking, swaying, or slow dancing is an excellent way to relax and distract yourself from labor pain. It stimulates mechanoreceptors in your brain, which decreases your pain perception. Incidentally, hugging, kissing, and hand-holding do the same thing. No wonder they feel so good!"
> —Judith

Movement and Your Baby's Position

The best birth position for your baby is occiput anterior (head down, with the back of the head against your belly). However, many babies assume an occiput posterior position (head down, with the back of the head against your back), which often results in a longer, more painful labor.

In the last weeks of pregnancy, your posture may affect your baby's position in your uterus. (Research on this is just beginning.) Semi-reclining may encourage your baby into a posterior position, so it's a good idea to avoid semi-reclining: Skip lounging on the couch, sleeping propped up with pillows, and kicking back in your chair at the office. If your car has bucket seats, straighten up your driving posture with a small pillow behind your back. When you're sitting in a chair, lean forward. Better yet, sit on a stool or a birth ball instead. Rest and sleep on your side.

If your baby is in a posterior position when labor starts, you'll probably feel your contractions as back pain. This happens because the back of your baby's head is pressing on

your spine. You may not get the relief between contractions that's typical in labor. Also, your labor may last longer because your baby needs to rotate more to fit under your pubic bone and needs more wiggle room to descend through your pelvis.

Movement and posture during labor are especially important with a posterior baby. You'll feel least comfortable on your back, because gravity will press your baby's head on your spine. (Actually, you'll feel least comfortable on your back regardless of your baby's position.[12]) Any position that widens your pelvis—such as climbing stairs two at a time, squatting, sitting on a birth ball, or kneeling on all fours with legs spread—will help your baby rotate and descend. If you have freedom of movement, you'll find yourself trying a variety of positions, searching for the one that feels best at the moment. Even if you don't find that perfect position, your movement will bring you some comfort.

Preventing Fatigue

Actively working with labor can be challenging and tiring. It's important to prevent fatigue so you can keep working with your labor for as long as it takes. Movement in labor doesn't mean endless hallway pacing, stair climbing, or floor washing. You could do all these things if you want to, but it's probably wiser to conserve your energy.

Here are a few ways you can stay active while your body is supported and relaxed:
- Rock in a comfortable rocking chair.
- Sit and sway on a birth ball.

- Bounce, rock, or sway while kneeling and leaning forward over a birth ball.
- Slow dance to music while your partner hugs and supports you.
- Lie on your side or sit in a tub of warm water. Because the water supports your entire body, you can easily

© Marilyn Nolt

roll from side to side, raise and lower your body, and move your limbs. The pressure and warmth decrease pain perception and increase circulation and oxygenation.

If you talk to friends who have given birth normally, you'll hear stories of labors spent dancing, doing pelvic rocks, stomping, squatting, or sitting on the toilet. Though each story will be unique, they'll all share the element of freedom—freedom to respond to each contraction in whatever way felt right. Partners, doulas, and caregivers can suggest specific movements and positions, but only you will know what helps you—and what helps you may change from moment to moment. That's why unrestricted mobility is so valuable.

CARE PRACTICE 3: CONTINUOUS EMOTIONAL AND PHYSICAL SUPPORT

Women, unlike other mammals, don't naturally labor alone. Why? Because our upright posture makes it more difficult for a baby to move through a woman's pelvis. The position changes that help our babies rotate and descend often require physical help. And in childbirth, as in many aspects of life, we humans do better when we're surrounded by those we trust, people who tell us we're doing well and encourage us forward.

Throughout time and across cultures, women have traditionally attended other women during labor and birth. Most births have happened at home, attended by community midwives. According to Sheila Kitzinger, "Woman to woman help in childbirth is the norm almost everywhere in the world."[13] The United States is one glaring exception. When U.S. birth moved from home to hospital, women lost the valuable support their ancestors had enjoyed—and their sisters in other countries continue to enjoy.

A 2003 review of studies including nearly thirteen thousand women found that compared to women who receive typical hospital care, women who receive continuous, one-to-one support throughout labor are:

- 26 percent less likely to have cesareans;
- 41 percent less likely to give birth with vacuum extractors or forceps;
- 28 percent less likely to use pain medications;
- 36 percent less likely to report dissatisfaction with their birth experiences.

Positive outcomes are more pronounced if support begins early in labor and is provided in settings where epidurals aren't routinely available. The study also suggests that results are better when support is provided by people present expressly to offer support, rather than hospital staff such as midwives or nurses.[14]

Modern hospitals make it difficult for staff to give birthing mothers continuous support. As birth has become more

medicalized, the focus of nurses' work has shifted from providing comfort to supervising medical interventions such as routine EFM, IV lines, epidurals, inductions, and cesareans. Although women expect their labor nurses to provide information, comfort, and support,[15] research shows that less than 5 percent of nurses' time is spent doing those activities.[16]

What Is Good Labor Support?

Good labor support is *not* watching the clock and checking IV lines and EFM printouts. It's making sure you're not disturbed, respecting the time that labor takes, and reminding you that you know how to birth your baby. Your helpers should spin a cocoon around you while you're in labor—create a space where you feel safe and secure and can do the hard work of labor without worry.

Good labor support can include reminding you to eat and drink, wiping your face, brushing your hair. It can mean helping you change position, putting a blanket around your shoulders when you're cold, taking it away when you're hot, whispering words of encouragement.

"My grandmother Nora always lit a candle in front of a statue of the Sacred Heart of Jesus when her daughters went into labor. Each candle stayed lit until the baby's birth. My mother and aunts knew that Nora was praying and caring for them, even if she was hundreds of miles away. My husband prayed the rosary over and over again as our daughter labored with her first baby. In New York City, Haitian grandmothers make a paste of papaya leaves and massage their daughters in labor. They also brew a special tea for strength and nourishment. Orthodox Jewish men recite ancient prayers as their wives labor. Family rituals like these support women in powerful ways."
—Judith

Good labor support can be your mother sitting in the corner, silently praying. It can be your partner holding your hand and reminding you what a great job you're doing. It can be your caregiver focusing complete attention on you as you cope with each contraction. Good labor support tries to respond to all your physical and emotional needs throughout labor.

Doulas Make a Difference

Who's a good candidate to support you during labor? You may want the familiar touch of your partner, your mother, or a close friend. You'll need someone you trust wholeheartedly, someone whose mere presence helps you relax. You'll also need someone who trusts birth, who won't be intimidated, and who won't lose self-confidence or confidence in you. That's a tall order.

A doula may fill any gaps you may have in your labor support team. In ancient Greece, doulas were important servants who helped their mistresses with all aspects of household management. Today, a doula is a woman trained to provide continuous physical, emotional, and informational support to a mother before, during, and just after she gives birth.

Doulas are well educated about birth, believe that birth is normal and natural, and have confidence in women's ability to give birth. A doula makes a point of getting to know you before your birth so she can provide better emotional and physical help. If you give birth in a hospital, she joins you, along with the other members of your labor support team.

Doulas don't replace the loving encouragement of your partner or the caring of your mother, sister, or friend. The special value of a doula is that she knows birth well. With her understanding of and strategies for nearly every situation, she can make the difference between being able to work with your labor and not being able to. Even more important is the quiet confidence she brings to your birth environment, which can help you and the other members of your support team feel relaxed enough to give your very best. Research has shown doulas to be so effective that neonatologist and researcher John Kennell says, "If a doula were a drug, it would be unethical *not* to use it."[17]

If you're interested in hiring a doula, ask your midwife, doctor, hospital, birth center, or childbirth educator for a referral. DONA International (formerly Doulas of North America) is an excellent resource for learning more about doulas and finding a doula in your community. (For more information on DONA International, see Appendix E or visit http://www.dona.org.)

It's important that you feel comfortable with your doula, and every good doula knows that. She'll expect you to want to get to know her before you decide whether to hire her.

CARE PRACTICE 4: NO ROUTINE INTERVENTIONS

Although research shows that routine and unnecessary interference in the natural process of labor and birth is not likely to be beneficial—and may indeed be harmful[18]—most U.S. births today are intervention-intensive. A majority of women surveyed for *Listening to Mothers* experienced the following interventions during labor:

- Continuous EFM (93 percent)
- Restrictions on eating (87 percent)

- IV fluids (86 percent)
- Restrictions on drinking (66 percent)
- Epidural anesthesia (63 percent)
- Artificially ruptured membranes (55 percent)
- Artificial oxytocin augmentation (53 percent)[19]

Common Practices You May Need to Question

Eating and Drinking Restrictions

Restricting oral intake is a long-standing obstetric tradition. It began in the 1940s, when women often gave birth under general anesthesia without airway protection. The rationale was that fasting reduces the chance of stomach contents entering the lungs (aspiration) in case of vomiting.

However, there's no evidence to support this belief.[20] Today epidural rather than general anesthesia is used when possible, which reduces the risk of vomiting and is safer for mother and baby. Also, airway protection is now standard medical practice for general anesthesia, so even if a patient does vomit under general anesthesia, the risk of aspiration is extremely small.[21] In other words: General anesthesia is rare in modern obstetrics, and aspiration is rare in modern general anesthesia. Furthermore, fasting doesn't guarantee an empty stomach, and clear liquids leave the stomach almost immediately. So really, there's no valid reason for tightly restricting eating and drinking in normal labor.

Various medical organizations have published sensible, evidence-based guidelines for oral intake during childbirth. The American Society of Anesthesiologists (ASA) and ACOG say women with no complications may be allowed to drink clear liquids during labor.[22] The American College of Nurse-Midwives (ACNM) recommends that healthy women experiencing normal labors determine appropriate intake for themselves.[23] The Society of Obstetricians and Gynaecologists of Canada (SOGC) states that "a woman in active labor should be offered a light or liquid diet."[24] The Cochrane Pregnancy and Childbirth Group recommends a low-residue, low-fat diet during labor.[25]

Despite all the evidence and advice to the contrary, many doctors and hospitals *still* restrict oral intake in labor. If your caregiver or birth site is one of these, labor at home—where you can eat and drink as needed—as long as possible.

Overall, we encourage you to eat and drink in labor if your body tells you to. If your labor is short and intense, you may not be hungry or thirsty. You probably will be if your labor is long, and you should eat and drink whatever appeals to you.

IV Fluids

IV fluids are used to prevent dehydration in women restricted from eating and drinking and to provide quick access to a vein in case of emergency. IV therapy has been a routine labor procedure since the late 1970s, but its value and safety are questionable.[26]

While an IV may lower the risk of dehydration in a woman who's truly unable to eat or drink in labor, it has drawbacks, too. It prevents her from moving freely, it may raise her stress level, it may cause fluid overload, and it doesn't ensure adequate nutrient and fluid balance for the demands of labor.[27] Because life-threatening emergencies and the need to restrict oral intake in laboring women are rare, research suggests that routine IV use is not likely to be beneficial.[28]

Continuous EFM

Your baby's heart rate can be monitored either continuously or intermittently, using any of the following devices:

- A **fetoscope** is a stethoscope with a large head designed for listening to fetal heartbeats.
- A **Doppler** is a hand-held ultrasound device that transmits fetal heartbeats to a speaker.
- **External EFM** is an ultrasound device held against a mother's abdomen with a belt. The belt is connected to a large machine that measures and records both contractions and fetal heartbeats.
- **Telemetry EFM** is a wireless version of external EFM.
- **Internal EFM** uses an electrode inserted in the baby's scalp to read his or her pulse and a catheter inserted in the uterus to detect pressure. These are connected by wires to a machine that measures and records contractions and fetal heartbeats.

Electronic fetal monitoring was introduced into obstetrics in the 1970s and quickly became standard practice for all hospital births, even though there was no research at the time to support its value for low-risk births. EFM does provide more information than a fetoscope or Doppler: It shows how contractions affect your baby's heart rate. But does this extra information lead to better outcomes?

A great deal of research done well after EFM was introduced compares fetoscope and Doppler use with continuous EFM. Evidence shows no difference in outcomes for babies and a higher rate of cesareans and operative vaginal deliveries for mothers with continuous EFM. Why? It's difficult to interpret EFM printouts. Misread printouts lead to mistaken conclusions, and caregivers often intervene unnecessarily when labor is actually progressing normally and baby is doing fine. In other words: For most labors, more intensive monitoring increases obstetric intervention (and risk) with no clear benefit for babies.[29]

Unfortunately, this evidence is largely ignored in U.S. birth. Most women are willing and happy to be closely monitored because they believe it makes birth safer for their babies. But continuous EFM not only increases the risk of cesarean with no benefit to babies, in most cases it also severely restricts maternal mobility. Unless telemetry is used, continuous EFM requires you to stay in bed and restricts your ability to change positions. It also restricts your access to comfort measures like a shower, bath, or birth ball. And despite your support team's best efforts, they'll probably find themselves focusing more on the monitor than on you, the one who's actually doing the work shown on the printout.

If you have a health complication, if you're given Pitocin, if you have an epidural, or if your baby is developing a problem, you'll need continuous EFM. Otherwise, intermittent monitoring with a stethoscope, a Doppler, or EFM is better. The ACOG supports both intermittent auscultation and EFM for women without complications.[30] The Association of Women's Health, Obstetric and Neonatal Nurses (AWHONN) recommends intermittent listening with a Doppler or fetoscope, rather than continuous EFM, for women with no complications.[31]

Speeding Up Labor Artificially

Speeding up labor may sound appealing, but research shows that routinely interfering with the pace and length of labor is not likely to be beneficial.[32] Each labor is unique; it's hard to say when a labor has gone on too long or not long enough. The length of your labor is influenced by many factors, including your baby's size and position, your confidence, your ability to move freely, your access to a variety of comfort measures, and the quality of your labor support.

There's strong evidence that breaking your water (manually rupturing your amniotic sac) will shorten your labor if your labor is prolonged or contractions are very slow, but it carries risks, too. When your membranes are broken manually, both you and your baby are exposed to greater risk of pressure injury as well as greater risk of infection. Research also shows an increase in cesareans with early rupture of membranes.[33]

Because having ruptured membranes for a long period of time raises your risk of infection, the medical clock starts ticking once your water breaks. If your labor doesn't progress rapidly, your caregiver will probably suggest artificial oxytocin (Pitocin) to speed things up. And then the cascade of interventions begins.

Current data doesn't show that liberal Pitocin use to speed up labor clearly benefits the women and babies receiving it.[34] It makes contractions stronger and harder to handle. It doesn't trigger endorphin release, which decreases pain perception. It also necessitates continuous EFM, an IV, and sometimes a bladder catheter. The stronger contractions, the loss of endorphins, the additional interventions, and the restricted mobility brought on by Pitocin all increase the possibility that you'll need an epidural—which carries risks of its own (see page 119).

A systematic review of the research suggests that only women with truly abnormal labor progress should have their water broken, and that only women with truly prolonged labors and sluggish uterine activity should receive Pitocin.[35] Neither intervention should be used routinely. According to the Cochrane Collaboration, letting women move around and eat and drink as they please may be at least as effective—and

certainly more pleasant—for many women who need augmentation.[36] In most cases, eating, drinking, urinating, and
movement can get a sluggish labor going.

Epidural Anesthesia and Analgesia

Most women fear childbirth pain and are eager to use pain
medication—especially epidurals, which are very effective
at relieving pain. In some hospitals over 90 percent of
laboring women have epidurals. Among the women surveyed
for *Listening to Mothers*, 63 percent reported having an
epidural, but when provided with four true statements about
side effects of epidurals, 26 to 41 percent of the women
surveyed were unsure whether to agree or disagree.[37]

If you have an epidural, your pelvic muscles relax and
don't offer the resistance your baby needs to rotate and
descend with each contraction. Since you have no need to
cope with pain naturally, your body may not get the signal
to keep labor going by releasing more oxytocin, and you
may need Pitocin. If you have an epidural, you'll require
continuous EFM, an IV, and possibly a bladder catheter.[38]
The changes in the physical process of birth and the interventions required to ensure safety during an epidural
introduce several risks.

Research clearly links epidurals with fewer normal
vaginal deliveries, more instrument deliveries, and longer
labors, particularly for first-time mothers. Women with
epidurals are more likely to have fever during labor, and
as a result, their babies are more likely to be evaluated and
treated for infection. This means mother and baby get
separated.[39] There's some evidence (though less conclusive)
that epidural use—especially by first-time mothers—increases
the risk of cesarean.[40]

You may be told that epidural medication does not
reach the baby. This isn't true: Baby gets it within seconds
of administration. There's increasing evidence that all
labor pain medications disturb newborn behaviors like
hand-to-mouth movements and sucking, which can harm
breastfeeding initiation.[41] Also, babies of medicated mothers
tend to cry longer and have higher temperatures than babies
of unmedicated mothers.[42]

We advise you to weigh the risks and benefits of epidurals carefully before deciding whether to have one. You'll want to consider your unique circumstances, too. For example, you or your baby may have a health problem that necessitates a cesarean, and an epidural is usually the best anesthesia for this surgery. Or your labor may be especially long and exhausting, in which case an epidural may give you a much-needed break.

If you can work actively with labor and if you have continuous emotional and physical support, you'll be less likely to need an epidural—or you'll need it later in your labor. Getting less epidural medication, getting it later in labor, and letting it wear off before you push go a long way toward reducing the risks of epidurals.

CARE PRACTICE 5: SPONTANEOUS PUSHING IN NON-SUPINE POSITIONS

When to Push

Many doctors and nurses discourage a woman from pushing until her cervix is completely dilated and/or encourage her to hold her breath and push without a natural urge once her cervix is fully dilated. There's no research to support these practices. Breath holding without the natural urge to do so is exhausting and deprives a baby of much-needed oxygen.

It's almost too obvious, isn't it? The signal that it's time to push is feeling the urge to push. If your baby is low in your pelvis, you may feel the urge to push before or at the time of full dilation. But if your baby is high in your pelvis at full dilation, you probably won't feel the urge to push until your baby's head moves well down in your pelvis. As your baby moves lower in your pelvis—especially when your baby's head touches your perineum (the tissue that forms the floor of your pelvis)—you'll find yourself involuntarily holding your breath during contractions. You may also naturally grunt and groan during pushing contractions.

How long will the pushing take? As long as it takes. Pushing shouldn't be limited as long as you and your baby are doing well. Like Silly Putty, your perineum takes time and effort to soften and stretch. Once it's soft and stretchy, your baby is easily born. Some caregivers interrupt this process and do an episiotomy (cut the perineum to enlarge the vaginal opening). Research shows that routine episiotomy is harmful.[43]

Pushing Positions

Throughout history and around the world, women have used both upright and gravity-neutral positions to push their babies out. They've often used objects like posts, ropes, and trees to get better leverage. They've also used birth supports or stools made from bricks, wood, or stone to help them squat, crouch, or kneel. Before birth forceps were invented in the 1600s, women were never shown giving birth on their backs.

Today more than 70 percent of American women give birth in supine positions (lying on their backs).[44] They're encouraged to give birth this way even though research shows it's harmful.[45] Lying on the back can lower a laboring woman's blood pressure, and the weight of her uterus on major blood vessels can reduce blood flow to her baby.

On the flip side, research supports traditional birth positions. Studies show that pushing in upright postures shortens the pushing stage and decreases the incidence of severe maternal pain and abnormal fetal heart rate.[46] Squatting widens the pelvic diameter, creating more room for the baby to descend.[47]

The best position for *your* birth is the one that's most comfortable for *you* at any given moment. By responding to what you feel, you make birth easier for you and your baby. You may change positions often, moving from kneeling upright to kneeling on all fours, or from standing to squatting. Or you may find yourself tightening and relaxing vaginal and perineal muscles as you sway from side to side or rock back and forth.

Using a variety of positions lets you respond to your baby's changing position as he or she descends, rotates, and extends in an effort to be born. Standing, kneeling, and squatting help gravity pull your baby down and protect your birth canal and baby from excessive pressure. Gravity-neutral positions—kneeling on all fours, side-lying, and semi-sitting—

are perfect for resting between contractions and may help you if you're exhausted.

If your baby enters your pelvis in the occiput posterior position (see page 109), kneeling on all fours takes the pressure of the back of your baby's head off your spine and may give your baby enough room to rotate to the occiput anterior position. Dangling in a supported squat, with a helper supporting you under your arms and with no weight on your legs or feet, lengthens your torso and allows your pelvis to move freely.

When it's time to push your baby out, remember that instinct, tradition, and science are all on your side. Current evidence shows that letting you assume whatever position you find most comfortable, encouraging you to push in response to what you feel, and letting you push as long as you and your baby are doing well are all beneficial practices.[48] AWHONN recommends that all pregnant women receive information about the benefits of upright positions and that nurses encourage squatting, semi-sitting, standing, and upright kneeling positions.[49]

CARE PRACTICE 6: NO SEPARATION OF MOTHER AND BABY, UNLIMITED OPPORTUNITY FOR BREASTFEEDING

Throughout most of human history, mothers and babies have stayed together from the moment of birth. Close to their mothers, babies stay warm and safe and can nurse frequently.

When U.S. births moved from home to hospital in the 1900s, for the first time in history mothers and newborns were routinely separated. Babies were kept in nurseries and brought to their mothers only for scheduled feedings. Mothers waited long hours to see and hold their babies, and often they didn't even see their newborns unclothed until they went home days or weeks after birth.

Recent research supports the traditional practice of keeping mothers and newborns together.[50] Evidence shows that this is a key element of nature's plan. Women experiencing normal birth have high levels of catecholamines, oxytocin, and endorphins. Catecholamines ensure that mother and baby are alert and ready to get to know each other. Oxytocin helps raise a mother's breast temperature and helps her feel calm and responsive.[51] As she holds her baby skin-to-skin, her baby's hand and head movements stimulate more oxytocin and endorphin release. The oxytocin helps her uterus stay contracted, which prevents excessive bleeding, and also increases milk production. The endorphins keep her calm and relaxed, and through her breast milk, they help her baby stay calm and relaxed, too.

Experts now recommend that right after birth, a healthy newborn should be placed skin-to-skin on the mother's abdomen or chest and should be dried and covered with warm blankets.[52] The mother's temperature adjusts naturally to keep her baby warm.[53] Newborns (including premature babies) held skin-to-skin by their mothers cry less and stay warmer than newborns placed in warming cribs.[54] Skin-to-skin contact also exposes babies to their mothers' normal bacteria instead of hospital germs, which lowers their risk of getting sick.[55]

Other benefits of skin-to-skin contact for newborns are easier, more regular breathing; higher, more stable blood sugar levels; and a natural progression to breastfeeding.[56] Most babies kept skin-to-skin with their mothers after birth instinctively crawl to the breast, latch on, and start nursing all by themselves. Even brief separation can interfere with their ability to do this.[57]

Any care that needs to be done immediately after birth can be done with your baby skin-to-skin on your chest, with a light, warmed blanket over you both. Weighing and measuring can be delayed for several hours. As midwife Ina May Gaskin says, you're entitled to "keep your prize."[58]

Chapter 9

FINDING COMFORT IN LABOR

We have a secret in our culture,
and it's not that birth is painful.
It's that women are strong.
—Laura Stavoe Harm

Having continuous emotional and physical support and being able to move in response to what you feel go a long way toward helping you find comfort during labor. But there's an array of additional simple comfort measures that can help you, too. This chapter explains what they are and how they work.

VIEW LABOR AS A TASK, NOT A TRIAL

One of the first—not to mention easiest—things you can do to bring comfort to your labor is to approach it with a positive attitude. View labor as an important job that only you can do, instead of an ordeal you must simply endure and would rather avoid.

Yes, labor is hard work, but hard work surely isn't new to you. It's a basic element of most women's lives; we put in long hours, hold demanding jobs, cram for exams, care for small children, and much more. And for many of us, leisure involves work, too: running, hiking, exercising at the gym, skiing, swimming.

The hard work of our daily lives is different from our great-grandmothers' work, but the work of labor and birth hasn't changed a bit over the years. Our great-grandmothers had to find ways to conserve strength and stay as comfortable as possible from one contraction to the next. So do we.

Here's some good news: This is work we innately know how to do, and we do it beautifully. Many of the comfort measures that helped our great-grandmothers and the generations of women before them still work well in labor and birth today. Women still reap the same great rewards for their efforts, too: satisfaction, confidence, empowerment, joy, and a new baby.

There's no way you can be *completely* comfortable in this work. But simply by searching for comfort—by accepting the job of working actively with your labor—you'll manage the pain of your contractions, keep labor going, and come out of labor richer in many ways.

CREATE A COMFORTABLE ENVIRONMENT

No matter what we're up to, we humans almost always feel better and do better in a safe environment—in a place safe from harm and threat, in a place safe from judgment and control, in a place where we're respected and cared for. For women in labor, this safe place is a private place.

Even though we (unlike other mammals) don't naturally give birth alone, we don't naturally give birth onstage either. As in other intimate and important activities, in labor we relax and focus better if we don't feel observed, evaluated, or interrupted.

If you are disturbed or feel observed, if you have to worry or think too deeply about what's going on around you, or if you're surrounded by unfamiliar and discouraging sights, sounds, smells, and people, your body launches a stress response. It releases large amounts of adrenaline to help you face what your brain perceives as a threat. The body gears up to either stand and fight the threat or turn and run to escape it.

Adrenaline tells your muscles to tense up, your senses to pay close attention, and your heart to pump blood rapidly to all parts of your body. You're suddenly on guard and ready for anything. If you've ever swerved or slammed your brakes while driving to avoid an accident, or tripped and caught yourself before falling, you know what a stress response feels like. That sort of tense anxiety can shut down labor or make it a lot more difficult.

The quest for safety in birth can be a double-edged sword. Most women choose to give birth in hospitals because they believe hospitals are the safest place to give birth. But ironically, hospitals are *not* safer than birth centers and homes for the great majority of births. (See pages 43 and 56.) And hospitals make it more difficult for birthing women to feel safe in the way they truly need.

If you're giving birth in a hospital, you'll need to plan for privacy, support, and a comfortable environment. You should consider hiring a doula, and you should stay at home for most of your labor. When you leave for the hospital, bring with you some sights and smells of home: your pillow, your own nightgown and clothes, a stuffed animal from your childhood, a picture of your family. At the hospital, create as much privacy as possible by shutting doors and restricting the comings and goings of staff.

No matter where you give birth, make it a comfort zone. Do simple things that always help you feel better. Labor is hard work, but it shouldn't be torture. To make sure it's not, be good to yourself and let others take care of you. For example, in early labor take a shower or a long, leisurely bath, shave your legs, wash your hair, get into comfortable clothes. As labor progresses, brushing your teeth and having your face washed or your hair brushed are great pick-me-ups. Urinating often helps you stay comfortable and helps keep labor progressing. Eating and drinking give you the energy you need to finish the journey.

REDUCE YOUR PAIN PERCEPTION

You already know a lot about pain; everyone experiences some degree of pain in life. You already know what to do about it, too: You either eliminate its cause or somehow reduce your perception of it. If you've ever walked, rocked, or moaned with menstrual cramps, or hobbled slowly with blisters from a new pair of shoes, you've had practice reducing your pain perception.

What you may not know is why such tactics work. Research has revealed many specific mental and physical factors that reduce pain perception, such as:

- Relaxation
- Movement
- Smell

- Distraction
- Temperature change

Pain messages travel to the brain on thinner nerves, and sensory messages on thicker nerves. Thicker nerves transmit information faster, so if a pain message and a sensory message are sent at the same time, the brain gets the sensory message first. That's why rubbing an ache (which sends a sensory message) eases the pain.

There are many ways you can use this knowledge to reduce your pain perception in labor. On the following pages, we'll give you ideas to get you started. Use them to create your own dance of rhythm, ritual, and relaxation. These "three Rs of childbirth" are a time-tested recipe for coping effectively with contractions.

Your Usual Tension Tamers

Are there certain things you do in daily life to reduce stress or take a break? Spend some time thinking about what helps you truly relax. These same things are likely to help you in early labor.

Maybe you're soothed by making a cup of tea—filling the kettle, waiting for the water to boil, adding the tea, letting

it steep, pouring the tea into a favorite mug, adding sugar and milk, and finally taking that first wonderful sip. Or perhaps you have a bath ritual—turning the hot water on, carefully adding bubble bath, waiting for the tub to fill, and then soaking luxuriously. Maybe you have a calming daydream—imagining your next vacation, seeing yourself at the beach, hearing the waves, smelling the sea, feeling the warm breeze.

Reading a book, watching TV, and listening to music are other common ways to relax. More active methods like taking long walks, dancing, and singing are popular, too. Even cleaning the house works for some people! Whatever your usual tension tamers may be, they're bound to work well in early labor. We recommend that you stay home and use them as long as they're effective.

As your labor progresses, getting comfortable and staying relaxed will be more challenging, and you may want to try some of the following methods. In preparation for childbirth, practice them when you're stressed out trying to make an appointment on time, when you're frustrated and stuck in traffic, or when you have a headache or a charley horse.

Conscious Breathing

Conscious breathing (especially slow breathing) reduces heart rate, anxiety, and pain perception. It works in part because when breathing becomes a focus, other sensations (such as labor pain) move to the edge of your awareness.

Conscious breathing is an especially useful labor tool because it not only keeps you and your baby well oxygenated, it's also easy to learn and use. It's naturally rhythmic and easy to incorporate into a ritual. And best of all, breathing is the one coping strategy that can't be taken away from you—even if you're stuck in bed attached to an electronic fetal monitor and intravenous fluids.

Conscious (or patterned) breathing used to be the hallmark of Lamaze childbirth education. It's not anymore (see page vi)—though some educators and caregivers think it still is. It's true that conscious breathing can help you relax and feel less pain during contractions. It's also true that there's no "right" way to breathe in labor, despite what others may tell you. Slow, deep breathing helps most women manage the pain of contractions. But the right way for *you* to breathe is whatever feels right to you. Issues like your number of breaths per minute, breathing through your nose or your mouth, or making sounds (like *hee-hee*) with your breaths are only important if they make a difference for you.

It may help you to have a visual focus to accompany your conscious breathing. You can recall an image with your eyes closed, focus on a picture or special object from home, keep your eyes on your partner, or simply stare at a spot on the wall. You may also find that as labor progresses, faster, shallower breathing—like a dog gently panting—feels better.

You'll figure out what works best for you. And what works best will probably change as you move through labor.

Tension Release

Most people don't know how physically tense they are from moment to moment. It's likely that you're usually a lot more tense than you think you are. Spend some time becoming more aware of body tension so you can practice consciously letting it go. Systematically tensing and then releasing specific body parts can increase your awareness of tension.

Childbirth educator, doula, and birth counselor Penny Simkin calls this the "roving body check."[1] Here's how to do it: Find a comfortable position in which your entire body is supported. Starting with your head and moving down to your toes, slowly tense and then release one body part at a time. You can also do this exercise with your labor partner. Your partner touches a part of your body, and you tense it. Then you release the tension.

The roving body check not only helps you identify physical tension, it also helps you learn to consciously release that tension. If you can consciously relax in labor, childbirth will seem more doable.

Music and Other Sounds

The sounds that surround you in labor are important. Some women need quiet, while others prefer noise of some kind. Sounds that create natural images—like running water, waves, birds, wind, or rain—often comfort and empower laboring women. So does music.

Listening to music is a simple and pleasant way to change your mood, forget your troubles, lighten your heart, and focus your mind. Music can fire you up or settle you down, inspire you or sadden you. As you move from one contraction to another in labor, music can relax you, energize you, or help you find a rhythm.

As you get ready for labor and birth, don't forget to prepare some music and something to play it on. Collect music that gets you going (perhaps Latin or African music, percussive music, or upbeat symphonic music) as well as music that helps you focus and settle down (perhaps chamber music, folk songs, choral works, or lullabies). When you put it to use, it'll get you instinctively moving, swaying, rocking, and opening up.

Whatever your sound preferences and wherever you give birth, you'll need to find a way to keep unwanted noises from distracting and disturbing you. Keep your door shut, turn off the ringer on your phone, unplug the TV—do whatever it takes to help you focus.

Heat and Cold

You'll probably find your body temperature fluctuating during labor. One minute you're shivering; the next you're hot enough to fling all your clothes off.

If you're cold, have someone warm a blanket for you. (At home, just toss the blanket in your clothes dryer for a few minutes.) Ask for a shawl or light sweater over your shoulders. Snuggle up with a hot water bottle or a heating pad. Fill a sock with uncooked rice and microwave it for three minutes; it'll provide moist heat for thirty minutes afterward.

If you're hot, shed some or all of your clothes. Have someone press a cold pack, a cold soda can, or a cool compress on your face, neck, and hands. If you're at a hospital, an ice-filled glove will bring quick relief.

Heat and cold are both pain relievers. If you have back pain, alternate heat and cold against your back. The temperature changes will reduce your pain perception by stimulating thermoreceptor sites in your brain.

Water

For most of us, a warm bath is more for relaxation than cleansing. The water massages our muscles to ease tension. It supports our bodies so we can change position easily. We feel weightless. It's easy to see why water is a friend to laboring women.

Some birthing women like the soothing sound and feel of water swishing in a bath. Others like the cleansing, rain-like sound and feel of a shower. In either form, water is a valuable way to reduce your pain perception, help you focus, and move your labor along. As you prepare for your baby's birth, make sure that a bathtub, shower, whirlpool, or birth pool will be available at your birth site.

Smell

Smell is a very powerful sense. When scents stimulate chemoreceptors in the brain, pain perception decreases. Scents can also trigger good or bad memories.

For most people, typical hospital smells are unfamiliar and associated with illness. Obviously, such smells aren't helpful for laboring women. In labor it helps to be surrounded with familiar and pleasant smells.

If you give birth in a hospital, wear your own clothes, bring your favorite pillow or blanket from home, and wear a fragrance you love. You may also want to have flowers, herbs, spices, essential oils, or other aromatic items that evoke good memories or bring pleasant images to mind. Doulas and midwives often use lavender and jasmine for laboring women.

Guided Imagery

We all daydream—we find ourselves unintentionally looking forward to vacations, reliving special family events, imagining our futures, and so on. Daydreaming frees you from an unpleasant reality, like a long commute, an all-night study session, or a sleepless night. When you mentally travel to another place or time, you recapture the joy or peace you found there once before.

You can take advantage of this in labor by using guided imagery to take you to a place where you feel peaceful, relaxed, and confident. The only difference between daydreams and guided imagery is planning where to go and how to get there. Will a picture, a smell, or a sound help you? Can you simply close your eyes and be there?

Guided imagery is also a good strategy to help labor progress. Imagining your cervix opening, your baby descending through your pelvis, and your baby nursing in your arms is an empowering way to cope with contractions. One woman recalls that during her first childbirth, her midwife suggested that she imagine her baby's first birthday.

Guided imagery is often more necessary at a hospital than at home. If you give birth in a hospital, you may find that home-based imagery works best to help you feel calm and confident.

Touch

Touch is an ancient comfort strategy. It eases pain as it conveys sympathy and understanding.[2] Sympathy and understanding are, of course, crucial for women in labor.

Comforting touch in labor is as simple as having a hand to hold, a shoulder to lean on, or arms to support you as you stand, squat, or kneel. It can be firm pressure in the right place on your aching back. It can be stroking your brow or brushing your hair off your face. It can be wiping your neck with a cool cloth as you slow dance with your partner. It can be supporting your shoulders as you sit on a birth ball.

Comforting touch can be massage. Hand and foot massage feels good, is relaxing, and may stimulate acupressure points that bring you pain relief. Shoulders tend to hold a lot of tension, and a massage there can help you release some of it.

Counterpressure is especially helpful if you have back labor. Firm pressure against your back with a fist, a cold soda can, or a tennis ball wherever it hurts the most (the spot changes as your baby rotates and descends) can relieve some of your pain.

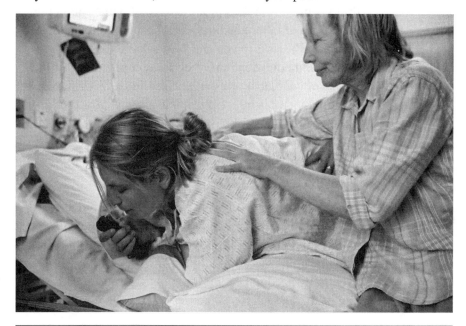

A rebozo (traditional Mexican shawl) can provide both pressure and support. A helper places the center of the rebozo against your back, forehead, belly, or whatever body part needs attention. Then he or she brings the ends around your body and pulls tightly. You can buy a rebozo from many online sources or simply use a large scarf or shawl. If you're in a hospital, you can use a sheet folded in half.

Touch doesn't have to be physical. It can be a blessing, like a mother lighting sacred candles while her daughter labors or an Orthodox Jewish man saying an ancient prayer as his wife gives birth. It can also be the vigilant watching, patient waiting, and complete attention of everyone who's with you.

What about Drugs?

Many people believe that normal birth means no medication. That's not always true. Drugs have appropriate uses, and they can help keep a difficult labor as normal as possible—especially when labor is very long and mother is exhausted. Women who labor in hospitals that restrict their ability to work actively with labor often find it very hard to manage without some medication.

However, it's important to know that *all* labor drugs—including the epidural—affect babies and alter the course of labor and birth. See Chapter 10 for ways to minimize the risks to you and your baby if you need drugs.

One "medication" that won't affect your baby or the course of your labor is a sterile water block.[3] A tiny amount of sterile water is injected just under the skin at four points on the lower back. The injection stings for a few minutes and then provides excellent relief of back pain for hours.

PACE YOURSELF

Although women worry most about the pain of labor, it's actually fatigue that often presents the greatest challenge. There's absolutely nothing you can do to change the pace or pattern of your contractions, and they do, of course, eventually need to become strong and powerful. But you *can* pace your activity to conserve strength and energy.

Assume you'll have a long labor. (If you don't, it'll be a pleasant surprise.) Alternate rest and activity throughout labor. In early labor, rest and conserve your energy as much as possible. In active labor, use supported positions and comfort strategies that don't use up all your strength. Remember to eat and drink; your body needs fuel for this journey.

FIND YOUR RHYTHM

At some point in labor, you'll "find your rhythm" or "get in a groove," much like a marathon runner does. You'll be living in the moment, doing without thinking.

To others you'll appear to be in another world. Your movements will be rhythmic; you'll relax between contractions; you'll respond to contractions in the same way over and over again, perhaps shaking your arms, rolling your head, breathing slowly, chanting, or praying. You'll be totally focused, but you won't necessarily look comfortable. You'll look like you're working very, very hard—which you are.

When this happens, you'll know endorphins are working their magic—dulling your pain and helping you ride your contractions intuitively. You'll be doing exactly what you need to do. You won't need to be rescued; in fact, the worst thing that could happen to you at this point is to be disturbed or interrupted. A healthy dose of encouragement, support, and respect are all you'll need from your support team.

GET REAL ABOUT LABOR PAIN

No matter how your labor unfolds or what comfort measures you use, you definitely won't feel like you're drifting off to sleep in a comfortable bed after a relaxing bath. (That comes later, with your baby in your arms!) But labor isn't meant to be hopeless, endless, lonely agony either.

Nature rewards you for working actively with labor. Strong, powerful contractions bring endorphin release and, with that, a measure of physical and emotional relief. Through your own efforts, you figure out what you need to do from one contraction to the next and you learn how to make the most of the time—however brief—between contractions.

Your support team helps you stay warm, cool off, save energy, move, and rest. Their words of encouragement keep you going.

It's realistic to expect that labor will be hard work, and it's also realistic to expect that you can do this work. Expect to be amazed at your own power and strength!

Chapter 10

CREATING A BIRTH PLAN AND BABY PLAN

Nothing happens unless first a dream.
—Carl Sandburg

The first step in making decisions and planning for your baby's birth is learning about the natural process of birth and about the choices you'll face. If you've read this book, gathered birth stories, and consulted other resources for information about normal birth, you've already taken this first step. You know what a healthy birth is, and you understand what helps birth as well as what hinders it.

This chapter is designed to help you take the next step. Naturally, we hope you'll decide to strive for normal birth. In other words, we hope you'll choose to pursue as natural a birth as is possible in your particular circumstances. This chapter will help you put that choice into action.

Many of the birth plans you may see in books or birth classes are simply checklists of medical procedures you do or don't want. To be truly useful, a birth plan should include much more. If you want to give birth normally, you'll need to develop strategies for making it happen. You'll also need to talk with your support team and your caregiver as your plans take shape. The more restrictive your birth site is, the more carefully you'll need to plan and the harder you'll have to work to keep your birth normal.

Remember, though, that your birth plan isn't an agenda. Creating a birth plan is like planning for a vacation. You read, talk to friends, and share ideas with your traveling companion. Together you sort through options and make some decisions. You settle on a beach vacation. You decide where and when to go. You make airline and hotel reservations. You know you want to rest, relax, and eat wonderful food, but you have no idea exactly how your vacation will unfold. You may eat every meal alfresco, take long walks on the beach, and watch breathtaking sunrises and sunsets. Or it might rain the whole time, so you might watch old movies, sleep late, read, and spend a lot of time in elegant restaurants. No matter how your vacation unfolds, you'll rest, relax, eat well, and have a wonderful time.

If you want to give birth normally, your planning should focus on creating an environment in which you feel safe enough to labor without worry and free enough to work with your unique labor. But as with a vacation, it's counterproductive to plan the details of birth too carefully. As poet Robert Burns says, "the best laid schemes o' mice and men" often go awry. Your labor may unfold differently than you expect. And you will probably respond to your labor in ways that feel right but aren't planned.

The following pages outline some key facts, options, and advice you might consider as you plan for your birth and the early days with your baby. In this chapter we summarize both the practices that help normal childbirth and the practices that hinder it. (For more information on these practices, see Chapter 8.) We also provide guidelines for appropriate use of interventions and suggestions for keeping birth as normal as possible if your labor and birth require medical intervention. Use them to create your own plans for birth and the early days with your baby.

Best Laid Schemes

Alicia had carefully planned and prepared for a natural vaginal birth after cesarean (VBAC), but circumstances challenged her to look beyond her birth plan, trust her body, and follow her instincts. Despite many interventions, Alicia and her helpers achieved their shared goal: keeping her labor and birth as normal as possible.

Alicia's Story

"My son Coby is one month old today. We just took a bath together, and he's calm and relaxed. I never thought of bathing with my older son, Ben, when he was a newborn, because I was still so sore from my cesarean. Every time I looked at my aching naked body, I resented how Ben's lovely labor had turned into an impersonal birth.

So I joined La Leche League and mothers' groups and became a doula and a Lamaze instructor. I was determined that women should feel supported and honored in birth. I got pregnant again just as we moved to Florida, far from my birth network. I turned to a birth center where the midwives were confident in my ability to have a normal birth.

At the end of my third trimester, I was feeling great but having a lot of Braxton-Hicks contractions that left me cranky and weepy. Before dawn one morning, I woke up with a sharp pain and couldn't get back to sleep. I went downstairs, made some pasta, and tried to relax on the couch. Then I lay in the tub for two hours listening to my relaxation tapes. By the time my husband, Phillip, woke up and joined me, the contractions were fairly close together and intense.

I kept in motion in my rocking chair and kneeling on all fours. We called my midwife, Debbie, and doula, Lorie, thinking things would continue to progress smoothly and quickly. Debbie asked if another midwife, Janice, could assist at my birth, too. Tears came to my eyes, I felt so cared for. Everything was just as it should be.

As Phillip, Ben, and I drove to the birth center, I listened to my tapes on a headset, feeling calm between contractions. At the birth center Ben happily ran into the play area, and Debbie and Lorie joined me in an examination room. Coby had dropped very low, which was great, but I was surprised to be only two centimeters open. My mucus plug had come loose at home, and I had fantasies of being six or seven centimeters after that nice bouncy car ride.

Debbie suggested we go to the beach and have lunch, but I wanted to rest. So I lay on the bed, and Lorie led me through relaxation exercises. Her voice was soothing, she had lavender in the air, and gentle music was playing. I spent a lot of time in the tub, then got out so an assistant could take my blood pressure and examine me. Lorie wanted me to move around to get Coby down more, so I did. She massaged me the whole time, until I insisted on going back to the tub.

I opened to five centimeters while floating in there, and I remember thinking, 'I've passed the point of last time's cesarean. I know I'll have a vaginal birth. My body has never been this open before. Coby is coming closer.'

Janice and her assistant, Colleen, appeared, and the birthing energy multiplied. I rolled around in the water most of the day, making noises and feeling confident that things were moving as they should.

Eventually my body started to push. It felt good, and I enjoyed thinking that I would have the water birth I wanted after a fairly easy labor. I kept vocalizing and floated on my side when the pushing got more intense.

I got out of the tub to pee, sat a bit on the birth ball, and then Debbie examined me on the birth stool. I hadn't progressed since the last exam, and my cervix was beginning to swell shut from the pushing. As powerful as the urge was, apparently I wasn't yet open enough. *[This is unusual, and you'll see why as Alicia's story unfolds. —Judith]*

Debbie said I had to stop pushing, and I got anxious and upset. It took all my effort and concentration to resist the urge. It was the hardest experience I've ever had. Everyone encouraged me as I wailed with each contraction. Women's hands were all over me, pressing relief into my hips and back, trying to help me relax and not push.

Later someone checked me, and the swelling had shrunk. I was at five centimeters again. But now a new hurdle appeared: meconium. The midwives quietly examined the chux pad, trying to decide if there was a lot or a little. They threw it away, then took it out of the garbage to look at it, then back in, then out again. Finally Janice said that as much as they didn't want to, we should go to the hospital.

Janice talked to me about there being many different ways to give birth. She explained that the meconium was not an emergency, but it meant we needed to be closer to my back-up doctor.

The whole crew came along (except tired little Ben, who had gone home with my parents). I knelt in the back of the minivan, with my head on my arms and my butt in the air. Lorie sat next to me, rubbing my back. We made it to the hospital and wormed our way through the halls and upstairs to labor and delivery.

We got admitted to a room, where I was monitored. Coby had turned in me, and I was opening a bit but was swollen again. I thought, 'Unless they let me stand on my head to relieve this pushing, my cervix is going to swell shut, and there will be nothing coming out of my vagina tonight.'

I decided to have an epidural. I didn't want to, but I didn't think I could make it without medicine. It wasn't the pain but resisting the urge to push that was horrible, and I desperately needed to rest.

As soon as the medicine took effect, I fell into a deep nap, waking myself up to make sure the monitor showed Coby was doing all right. Lorie assured me she was watching things. Every once in a while she had me roll onto my side, where Coby was happier.

Then labor stopped, so on came the Pitocin. I continued to dilate, tremble, and doze. I remember waking and thinking, 'I've never been here before. I'm really doing it. It's going to happen; it really is.'

Coby was working his way down, and I was fully dilated. It was time to push. Janice gave me homeopathic herbs, and I swigged some Gatorade to boost my energy. My VBAC-friendly doctor came in. I pushed and pushed, but I couldn't feel the urge because my epidural was so strong. They turned it down, and then I could feel Coby's head inside me. I asked for a mirror to watch. The nurses were supportive and confident I'd have my vaginal delivery. When they couldn't find a delivery room mirror, one nurse ripped a mirror off the bathroom wall, hooks and all.

It was hard to push without the strong urge I'd gotten used to feeling, and the doctor had to use a vacuum extractor for a few pushes. I watched Coby's head come out. The cord was wrapped so tightly around his neck that it couldn't be loosened, so the doctor cut it and quickly helped me deliver the rest of Coby's body. His tight, short umbilical cord explained a lot: his slowed heart rate, his stress-induced meconium, and his inability to come down any further. *[It also explains Alicia's cervical swelling. Though Coby was low in her pelvis, rapid labor might have caused him distress. Alicia's body prevented him from moving too fast. —Judith]*

Coby had gotten bumped around quite a bit, and the staff wanted to check him out before giving him to me. They held him up, all naked and gooey, like a curly caterpillar, and I thought, 'Maybe I can take him!' as I held my arms out. But they whisked him to the side of the room. They suctioned out the meconium he'd swallowed. When I heard him sputtering and breathing, I knew he would be fine.

Phillip was gaping over him, never having seen this kind of thing. I kept calling to Coby, and telling Phillip to talk to Coby. Coby looked right up at his dad when he heard his voice.

My placenta was hanging on for dear life and didn't want to come loose. So I did some nipple stimulation, and Janice jiggled it free.

As soon as Coby was stable, the hospital staff gave him to me and left. Janice encouraged me to nurse him right away. He latched right on—it was so simple, so natural, so normal. He weighed seven pounds at birth, just like Ben, who'd had the same cord situation. But this time I'd birthed with people who protected me, supported me, and encouraged me, and it made a big difference.

Even though I'd spent a lot of time planning for a smooth labor, Coby's birth ended up requiring considerable intervention. The next day I started to feel bad about my crazy labor and how technical it ended up becoming.

> But in retrospect, I think everything happened as it should. Coby and I are healthy because of the exceptional care and wisdom of my midwives. Going to the hospital when we did and having an epidural allowed me to have a lovely VBAC and feel great the next day. I was tired, but elated and in love with my husband and both my beautiful sons. I did it, and I am blessed."

PLANNING FOR NORMAL BIRTH

What Helps Labor

A good birth plan addresses the ways you'll help your labor along. This is the most important part of your birth plan. Regardless of the path your labor takes, how will you develop and maintain confidence in your ability to give birth? How will you find comfort and cope with contractions? What support will you need, and who will provide it?

Confidence

You'll surely discover a lot of ways to be confident on your own, but here are some ideas from other women to get you started:

- Talk with women who've had satisfying births.
- Read Chapter 7.
- Watch videos of natural birth, such as *Celebrate Birth!*, *Gentle Birth Choices, Open Minds to Birth*, and *The Timeless Way*. (You can expect to see these and other videos in your childbirth class. For more information on these and other videos, see Recommended Resources.)
- Recite and think about the birth affirmations below.
- Stay away from anyone who makes you frightened about birth.
- Read the book *Ina May's Guide to Childbirth*. (For more information, see Recommended Resources.)
- Talk to women who've given birth at home or at birth centers.

Birth Affirmations
- My body knows how to give birth.
- I'm strong and powerful.
- I'm surrounded by people who care about me.
- The work I'm doing is important.
- Women have been doing this work forever.
- The existence of birth technology doesn't mean I can't give birth safely without it.

Comfort

You aren't meant to suffer in labor. Nature intends that you respond to your contractions, not lie passively and feel tortured by them. As with other types of pain in your life, you should try to relieve labor pain in a variety of ways until you find something that works. Following are just some of the many comfort strategies you can try. (See Chapter 9 for more.)

- Move to ease your discomfort.
- Listen to music.
- Relax in a bath or shower.
- Get a hand or foot massage.
- Walk.
- Rock.
- Try some guided imagery.
- Sit and sway on a birth ball.
- Slow dance with or without a partner.
- Eat or drink when you're hungry or thirsty.
- Stay home as long as you feel comfortable there.
- Have your hair brushed.
- Sip tea.
- Keep your lips moist with lip balm.
- Brush your teeth every few hours.
- Have your face and neck wiped with cool water.
- Use a warm rice sock (see page 131) on your neck or lower back or under your belly.
- Stay active.
- Sit on the toilet.
- Change positions often.
- Breathe slowly.
- Moan with contractions.
- Pray.
- Push when your body tells you to.
- Use medication wisely.

Take some time to think about what might work well for you. But keep in mind that when labor is underway, you may find yourself responding to your contractions in ways you couldn't have imagined, tapping into a wisdom you didn't know you had.

Support

Research shows that labor is easier and birth outcomes are better if women receive continuous emotional and physical support.[1] Most women give birth in hospitals and expect doctors and nurses to provide this support. But in reality they see little of either, and when hospital staff are present, they're usually attending to or watching for complications, not comfort needs.

Regardless of where you give birth, you'll need minute-to-minute support. The following are just some of the ways you can plan for support:

- Have your partner attend childbirth classes with you.
- Tell your partner that his or her presence at birth is very important to you.
- Read *The Doula Book*. (For more information, see Recommended Resources.)
- Interview doulas and hire one who suits you.
- Ask your mother, your sister, or a close friend to be with you in labor.
- Tell your helpers that you want company at all times during labor and birth.
- Let your caregiver and support team know what kind of support you want, such as encouragement, comfort measures, help with changing positions, and advocating for you with hospital staff.
- Don't be afraid to ask nurses for help with non-medical needs.
- Stay at home, where support is easier to get, as long as you can.

What Hinders Labor

Many common medical interventions can hinder the process of birth by prolonging labor, discouraging you, and interfering with your ability to find comfort. These interventions can certainly be beneficial if they're used appropriately, when complications develop or the risk for complications is high. But they're often used inappropriately on healthy women whose labors are progressing normally. (See Chapter 8 for more details.)

To avoid interventions that hinder labor, you'll need some basic knowledge about their appropriate use and strategies for preventing inappropriate use. You'll also need to know how you can minimize the negative effects of truly necessary interventions and keep your labor as normal as possible. The following pages give you key information and suggestions to consider.

Continuous Electronic Fetal Monitoring (EFM)

What to Know
- Routine continuous EFM provides no benefit for babies and increases the risk of cesarean for mothers.[2]
- The American College of Obstetricians and Gynecologists (ACOG) says either intermittent auscultation or EFM may be used for healthy, low-risk women (almost all women). With auscultation, fetal heart rate should be monitored every thirty minutes in active labor and every fifteen minutes during pushing.
- The World Heath Organization (WHO) encourages intermittent manual listening and warns that EFM is often used inappropriately.

You'll need continuous EFM if:
- Your labor is induced or speeded up with Pitocin.
- You have an epidural.
- Your baby's heart rate changes.
- You or your baby has a health problem.

How to Avoid Unnecessary Use
- Remember that routine use of continuous EFM doesn't make labor safer for your baby.
- Find a caregiver who doesn't use continuous EFM routinely.
- Talk to your caregiver about intermittent fetal monitoring.
- Stay at home as long as possible in labor.

How to Keep Labor as Normal as Possible If You Need EFM

- Remember that your body knows how to protect your baby during labor.
- Continue to move as much as possible, both in and out of bed.
- Ask staff to turn off the monitor's sound.
- Ask staff to turn the monitor away from you and your helpers so it doesn't distract you.
- Ask to be disconnected from the monitor for regular trips to the toilet.
- Remind your helpers that *you* are the one in labor, not the machine.

Routine Intravenous (IV) Fluids and Oral Intake Restriction

What to Know

- Routine IV use restricts movement, decreases confidence, may over-hydrate mothers, and may contribute to low blood sugar in newborns.
- Restricting eating and drinking in labor depletes a woman's energy when she needs it most.[3]
- The WHO recommends offering women fluids by mouth and eliminating routine IV use during labor.
- The American Society of Anesthesiologists (ASA) recommends that low-risk laboring women be allowed to drink clear liquids (such as water, juice, carbonated drinks, clear tea, and black coffee).[4]

You'll need an IV if:

- You develop health problems or complications before or during labor.
- You're at high risk for complications.
- Your labor is induced or speeded up with Pitocin.
- You have an epidural.

How to Avoid Unnecessary Use

- Choose your caregiver and birth site carefully.

- Talk to your caregiver about your desire to eat, drink, and avoid unnecessary IV use.
- Confidently eat and drink while you labor at home.
- Labor at home as long as possible.

How to Keep Labor as Normal as Possible If You Need an IV
- Labor at home as long as possible.
- Eat and drink as your body commands while you're at home.
- Suck on ice chips, Popsicles, or lollipops during labor.
- Walk around with your IV pole.
- Stay as active as possible.
- Remember that you don't need the IV to have a safe birth and a healthy baby.

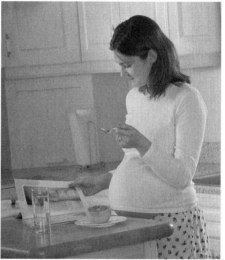

Movement Restrictions

What to Know
- Research shows that restricting movement reduces the effectiveness of contractions, prolongs labor, and increases Pitocin use.[5]
- The WHO encourages freedom of position and movement and discourages the supine (back-lying) position during labor.
- The ACOG encourages women to change position often.

You'll need to stay in bed or have help moving if:
- You're having preterm labor.
- You have severe pregnancy-induced hypertension.
- You have epidural or spinal medication.
- You have narcotic medication through an IV.

How to Avoid Unnecessary Use
- Discuss movement with your caregiver.
- Find out if your birth site restricts walking and movement during labor.

- Consider changing your birth site if it will restrict your movement.
- Labor at home as long as possible, walking and moving freely.
- Remember that walking, moving, and changing positions help your labor progress.

**How to Keep Labor as Normal as Possible
If Your Movement Is Restricted**
- Labor at home as long as possible, walking, moving, and changing positions freely.
- Change positions often in bed:
  - Move from side to side.
  - Sit on the side of the bed.
  - Kneel while leaning your head and shoulders against the raised head of the bed.
  - Lie in different directions; for example, move your head to the foot of the bed.
  - Squat while supported.
- Remember that the more you move, the more efficient your contractions will be.

Artificial Rupture of Membranes

What to Know
- An intact amniotic sac protects your baby's head and your vagina during labor.
- Artificially rupturing the sac increases your risk of infection and interventions (Pitocin, EFM, IV, restricted movement, and cesarean).
- Research shows that movement and hydration are often all that's needed to get a slow labor moving and that membranes shouldn't be ruptured routinely.[6]

You may benefit from having your water broken if:
  - Your labor is very difficult or slow to progress.

How to Avoid Unnecessary Use
- Discuss this intervention with your caregiver.

- Tell your caregiver that a longer labor is okay with you.
- Labor at home as long as possible.

How to Keep Labor as Normal as Possible
If Your Membranes Are Ruptured Artificially

- Be prepared for stronger contractions.
- Continue to use all the support and comfort resources you have.
- Keep moving and changing position often.
- Remember that your body knows how to birth your baby.

Directed Pushing

What to Know

- Research shows that routine directed pushing, breath holding, and limiting pushing during labor are not beneficial, and that prolonged breath holding may reduce fetal oxygenation.[7]
- The WHO recommends *not* directing laboring women to hold their breath or consciously sustain pushing.
- The American College of Nurse Midwives (ACNM) and the Association of Women's Health, Obstetric and Neonatal Nurses (AWHONN) recommend that a laboring woman's body direct any pushing.

Directed pushing may help you if:

- You've had an epidural and don't feel the urge to push.

How to Avoid Unnecessary Use

- Remember that your body knows how to push your baby out.
- Listen to and follow your body's signals.
- Change position often while you're pushing.
- Ask your helpers to support your efforts to push naturally.
- Be patient with your body.
- Visualize your baby rotating and descending through your birth canal.
- Ask your helpers to keep comforting you while you push your baby out.

- If you have an epidural, "labor down"—rest until you feel an urge to push.

How to Keep Labor as Normal as Possible
If You Use Directed Pushing
- Remember that your body knows how to birth your baby.
- Don't hold your breath for more than six seconds at a time.
- Push in an upright position.
- Rest between contractions.
- Be patient.
- Visualize your baby rotating and descending.
- Ask your helpers to keep supporting and comforting you.

Induction or Augmentation with Pitocin

What to Know
- Pitocin increases stress on your baby and your uterus and makes contractions more difficult to manage.
- Pitocin use necessitates an IV and continuous EFM, restricts your mobility, and raises your risk of epidural and cesarean.
- The WHO believes that Pitocin induction and augmentation are often used inappropriately.
- The ACOG notes the risks of Pitocin use and recommends cautious decision making.

You'll need induction if:
- Your labor is slow and doesn't respond to movement, position change, and hydration.
- You don't go into labor spontaneously by forty-two weeks gestation.
- You have a uterine infection.
- You have severe pregnancy-induced hypertension.
- Your baby has a growth problem.

How to Avoid Unnecessary Use
- Be patient waiting for labor to begin and to progress.
- Remember that your body knows how to give birth.
- Surround yourself with helpers who trust birth.

- Stay confident.
- Use all the comfort measures you've learned.
- Don't agree to be induced because your caregiver says your baby is getting too big.
- If your water breaks before contractions start, or if you're approaching forty-two weeks, discuss with your caregiver natural ways to stimulate contractions, such as drinking a bit of castor oil in juice, lovemaking, stimulating your nipples, and being active.
- Ask, "What if I wait?" if your caregiver is insistent about inducing labor.

How to Keep Induced Labor as Normal as Possible
- Make sure your helpers give you continuous emotional and physical support.
- Actively seek comfort in response to the pain of contractions.
- Remember that your body knows how to give birth.
- Visualize your baby rotating and descending through your birth canal.
- Keep moving and changing positions as much as possible.

Epidural Anesthesia and Analgesia

What to Know
- Seeking relief from labor pain without drugs protects your baby and your body from injury, helps labor progress, and facilitates breastfeeding, bonding, and other postpartum adjustments.
- Epidural use necessitates an IV, continuous EFM, and restricted mobility, and it relaxes vaginal muscles. All of these factors can prolong labor.[8]
- Epidural use increases the risk of instrument delivery and may increase the risk of cesarean.[9]
- Epidural use raises the risk of fever and postpartum separation to rule out infection.[10] Epidural drugs do reach your baby. Both of these factors can make breastfeeding initiation harder.

You may need an epidural if:
- Your labor is very long and difficult and you need to rest.
- You have a cesarean.
- Your blood pressure is very high.
- You don't have good labor support.
- Your birth site restricts your ability to find comfort in other ways.
- You can't move beyond your fear of labor pain.

How to Avoid Unnecessary Use
- Labor at home as long as possible.
- Choose your caregiver and birth site carefully.
- Discuss your desires with your caregiver.
- Make sure you have excellent labor support.
- Use all the non-drug comfort measures you can.
- Be patient and remember that your body knows how to give birth.

How to Keep Labor as Normal as Possible If You Have an Epidural
- Use a wide variety of other comfort measures for as long as possible, so you don't need an epidural for your entire labor.
- Wait to push until you feel an urge to do so ("labor down").
- Ask your helpers to massage your hands and feet and help you stay as active as possible.
- Be patient with your breastfeeding baby and spend as much skin-to-skin time together as possible.
- If your baby doesn't latch well at first or you have other breastfeeding problems because of your epidural, ask hospital staff (preferably a lactation consultant) to help you express colostrum and feed it with a small cup or eyedropper.
- To avoid aggravating breastfeeding problems, tell the hospital staff not to feed your baby formula or use bottles or pacifiers.

Episiotomy

What to Know

- Research provides no evidence that an episiotomy reduces the risk of perineal injury, improves perineal healing, prevents birth injury to babies, or reduces the risk of future incontinence. Rather, the evidence shows that routine or liberal use of episiotomy is likely to be ineffective or harmful.[11]
- The WHO recommends eliminating routine or liberal episiotomy.

You may need an episiotomy if:

- You or your baby is in distress.
- Your baby is very large or in an unusual position.

How to Avoid Unnecessary Use

- Ask potential caregivers their thoughts about episiotomy and choose your caregiver carefully.
- Push in upright positions that let your perineum stretch gently as your baby descends.
- Change positions often while you're pushing.
- Push spontaneously, according to your body's signals, not in a directed way.
- Remember that your body knows how to give birth.
- Be patient with your body.

Kegel Exercises

Your perineal muscles support your uterus and other organs like a hammock. Kegel exercises strengthen these muscles and are important for all women to do. If you have an episiotomy, Kegels increase circulation, decrease swelling, and help healing. Here's how to do a Kegel:

1. Get in any position: sitting, standing, or lying down.
2. Focus on the muscles around your urethra and vagina, not the muscles of your buttocks, thighs, or abdomen.
3. Tighten (contract) your perineal muscles as if you were trying to stop urinating. It should feel like you're lifting them.
4. Hold this contraction as tightly as you can for a slow count of ten. Don't hold your breath. As you master this exercise, increase your count to twenty.
5. Repeat ten times throughout the day.

What You Can Do If You Have an Episiotomy

- After birth, start doing Kegel exercises as soon as possible to help heal and strengthen your perineal muscles. (See the sidebar on page 153.)
- After birth, take warm baths to increase circulation and decrease pain and apply ice to reduce swelling.

Cesarean Surgery

What to Know

- Though some obstetricians tout the safety of cesareans and their value in preventing perineal damage, a systematic review of current research shows that vaginal birth is safer for mother and baby than a cesarean—unless there's a clear, compelling health reason for having a cesarean.[12]
- The risk of perineal damage in vaginal birth is extremely small if forceps, vacuum extractor, and episiotomy aren't used.
- Cesarean surgery increases your short-term risk of blood clots, stroke, surgical injury, infection, pain, separation from your baby, psychological trauma, longer hospital stay, emergency hysterectomy, and death. In the long term, it increases your risk of pelvic pain, bowel obstruction, infertility, and future pregnancy problems like ectopic pregnancy (pregnancy outside the uterus), placenta previa (placenta over the cervix), and uterine rupture.
- A cesarean raises your baby's risk of surgical injury, respiratory problems, and breastfeeding difficulties. It increases your future babies' risk of stillbirth, low birth weight, preterm birth, and central nervous system injury.
- If you've had a previous cesarean, there's a small chance your uterine scar could separate during labor and a small chance that the separation could endanger you or your baby. This is more likely if your labor is induced or if your scar is high and vertical.

You'll need a cesarean if:

- You are hemorrhaging.
- Your baby's oxygen supply is blocked.

- You have placenta previa.
- Your baby is in a transverse position (lying horizontally across your pelvis).
- You have poorly controlled diabetes or severe pregnancy-induced hypertension.
- You've had a previous cesarean, and your caregiver is unwilling to attend a VBAC or your hospital doesn't have round-the-clock anesthesia services.
- Your labor is not progressing at all, and either you or your baby is not doing well.
- Your baby is in a breech position (head up, feet or buttocks down) and your caregiver isn't skilled at assisting vaginal breech birth.
- Your baby's heart rate slows and doesn't improve when you change position, drink more fluids, breathe some oxygen, or turn your Pitocin down or off.
- You're carrying more than one baby, and one of your babies is in a transverse position or your caregiver isn't skilled at assisting vaginal multiple births.

How to Avoid Unnecessary Use

- Let your labor start and progress on its own unless there are clear, compelling health reasons to induce or speed up labor.
- Visit the Maternity Center Association (MCA) website (http://www.maternitywise.org). Download the free booklet *What Every Pregnant Woman Needs to Know about Cesarean Section* and read it.
- Discuss intermittent fetal monitoring with your caregiver.
- Remember that your body knows how to give birth.
- Plan for excellent labor support.
- Move and change positions often during labor.
- Labor at home for as long as possible.
- Work actively with your contractions.
- Keep up your energy by eating and drinking.
- Try lots of non-drug comfort measures before considering an epidural.
- If you have an epidural, let it wear off before pushing ("labor down").

- If you've had a previous cesarean, visit the MCA web page "Should I Choose VBAC or Repeat C-Section?" (http://maternitywise.org/mw/topics/vbac-cesarean). Choose a caregiver who supports your decision to have a VBAC.
- If your baby is breech, discuss external version (manually turning your baby head-down) with your caregiver.

How to Keep Birth as Normal as Possible
If You Have a Cesarean

- Have your partner and doula (or other helper) in the operating room.
- Hold your baby skin-to-skin as soon as possible after birth.
- Nurse your baby in the first hour after birth.
- Room in with your baby at the hospital.
- Have support from family and friends while you're in the hospital.
- Be patient with your baby as he or she learns to breastfeed.
- If your baby doesn't latch well at first or you have other breastfeeding problems, ask hospital staff to help you express colostrum and feed it with a small cup or eyedropper.
- To avoid aggravating breastfeeding problems, tell staff not to feed your baby formula or use bottles or pacifiers.

Learning from Experience

Sheila is planning for her second birth by examining what worked for her the first time and what didn't. She has more confidence this time, and she has a much clearer understanding of what *she* needs to cope with labor.

Sheila's Story

"As my second birth approaches, my anticipation is dominated by the question *What can I do differently this time to make it better?*

My first birth was by no means bad. In fact, it went well in many ways: a vaginal delivery, a simple twenty-minute pushing stage, no episiotomy or tearing, and a beautiful, healthy, eight pound nine ounce baby girl. But labor was long: eighteen hours from the rupture of my membranes (8:00 A.M.) to my first contraction (2:00 A.M. the next day)—during which period I got very little rest—and nineteen hours from there to delivery (9:00 P.M.). This culminated in my choosing an epidural for pain relief late in labor, something I'd committed myself to avoiding.

I gave birth with a midwife in a hospital comparatively supportive of natural childbirth. A hospital, however, is a hospital, and the staff couldn't overlook the fact that my membranes had already been ruptured for twenty-four hours when we arrived at 7:30 A.M. (The evening before, I'd refused admission and sedation to help me recharge for the work ahead.) Intermittent EFM and IV antibiotics were required.

My contractions had been coming quite regularly five minutes apart for a full hour before we left for the hospital, but they became erratic once we got there. I was just one centimeter dilated. After a couple of hours of erratic contractions, my midwife recommended Pitocin to get things moving better. I was too busy doing the work of labor to argue, so my husband stepped in and insisted that since the baby was fine, we should wait awhile and give the contractions time to pick up. She agreed, and sure enough, contractions were close, regular, and progressing within an hour. It was now 11:30 A.M.

As my contractions escalated, I finally understood why I'd read so much about the need for freedom of movement. I found myself responding and adapting to the pain actively and unconsciously, guided by something beyond reason. For one series of contractions, what made sense was to push against the wall. Then suddenly I would shift to crouching on the ground. Then I'd rock in the rocking chair. This dance went on and on.

I knew I was doing a 'good job'—managing the pain, living through it. It was as bad as I'd imagined, but I still had fight within. This confidence was based on the assumption that my cervix was dilating quickly.

But it wasn't. My midwife and nurses, to their credit, were reluctant to check my dilation often, but at this point they did so at my request. I was at three centimeters.

As the contractions grew more and more intense and coping with them became all-consuming, time flew by. I'd feel as though five minutes had passed, then look at the clock to find that more than an hour had. Day blurred into dusk, and I felt myself losing control, feeling frantic, tensing my entire body with each contraction, holding my breath.

There was room in my mind for almost nothing else but the unbelievable physicality of each moment. But in some pocket of mental clarity, I knew that my ability to handle the pain had changed because the pain itself had changed. It was stronger, sharper, faster, harder. That meant that I was making progress, opening up, getting closer to the end.

I knew that to keep going, I needed a shot of encouragement—not the kind I was already getting from my husband, midwife, and nurses, but *evidence* to support my conviction. I needed to hear that I was almost fully dilated, that all the work I'd been doing had helped. So I asked my midwife to check me. She was reluctant, but I prevailed.

I was so certain that she was going to announce, 'You're at seven!' When she said, 'Three and a half,' I collapsed into bed. I looked at the clock: I'd dilated just a half-centimeter in four hours. Every ounce of will to go on seeped out of me.

At that moment, I realized, 'I don't have to do this anymore.' I decided I wanted and needed pain relief. No one had even suggested it; my nurses, midwife, and husband had been absolutely supportive of unmedicated labor. When I told my midwife I wanted to discuss pain relief, she discouraged having an epidural. But I knew my problem was sheer exhaustion. It was 4:30 P.M., and I'd been awake for over thirty-two hours.

My husband, knowing the snowball effect an epidural can have, said, 'I know you can do this.' But to me, it wasn't a question of my ability. I'd been doing it for an eternity, and it had gotten me almost nowhere. I'd reached the end of my rope. I decided to go ahead with the epidural. Moments later, the anesthesiologist came in. Almost immediately, the drugs took effect and I fell into a two-hour sleep. It was 5:00 P.M.

Contractions slowed during my nap. When I awoke at 7:00 P.M., my baby's head still wasn't engaged. My midwife suggested nipple stimulation and brought in a breast pump to help. After a while, she checked my dilation. Seven centimeters—progress! Then a nurse suggested emptying my bladder—perhaps that was obstructing the head. It seemed to do the trick. A few minutes later, my midwife checked me again: ten centimeters, and the baby's head was engaged.

It was 8:30 P.M. and time to push. After all that had come before, I anticipated a long pushing stage. But twenty minutes later, after only a few contractions, our daughter Maisie emerged into the world.

What will I do differently this time around? I can't predict how labor will start or how long it'll take. I can't will my water not to break eighteen hours before contractions start. But I now know what I can do, say, think, and hear that'll help me manage labor better, both physically and emotionally.

I now know, for example, that it's critical to get as much rest as I can while I can. I think this will be easier this time simply because I'm no longer anticipating the unknown. With Maisie I was so excited and afraid and antsy that I couldn't possibly sleep. It was like I was five years old, waiting for dawn on Christmas morning. This time, if events unfold in the same way, I know I'll be much calmer.

I also know for sure now that I *will* survive labor, that my body *can* handle it from start to finish, and that it really will end at some point. In the thick of my first labor, when the pain was at its worst, I was sure of none of these things.

I now know that I need to focus on relaxing as much of my body as possible during a contraction, rather than tensing as I did during the toughest contractions with Maisie. I knew that intellectually going into my first labor, but that knowledge was of no use without knowing exactly what contractions would feel like.

I now know what I need to hear when labor gets really hard. 'You're *not* going to die.' 'This isn't going to last forever.' 'Your body can do this.' 'You've done this before.' I've asked my husband to tell me these things.

I now know that being in a standard hospital maternity room affected my confidence. As supportive as my midwife and nurses all were, we were in the same room and with the same staff I'd have had if I'd gone in intending to have an epidural and lie in bed for the duration of my labor. This time I'll give birth in an alternative birth center within a hospital—entirely separate from the regular maternity ward—with suites that have birth tubs, birth balls, and queen-size family beds. I think being in an environment that promotes natural, normal childbirth will make a big difference in my confidence.

As I sit a month from my due date, I'm more anxious than I was in my first pregnancy because I know in a visceral way what labor entails. But it's a completely different kind of anxiety, one that has empowered me to prepare in a more practical way for the task ahead.

Postscript

All my planning and preparation—both physical and psychological—paid off in the birth of my second daughter. Ellen Virginia was born underwater, into an environment of absolute tranquility, after just five hours of labor and about ten minutes of pushing.

Throughout each stage, I was able to maintain control, stay on top of the pain, and take things one contraction at a time. The water provided tremendous physical relief and, I am convinced, sped up the process substantially: I was five centimeters when I got in the tub and was ready to push twenty minutes later. Transition was barely detectable.

The warm water's effect on my pain was instantaneous. The moment I sank in the tub, I felt transformed. Though the pain certainly didn't disappear, it became both muted and more focused. The isolation of the pain helped me manage it. Rather than tensing up when a contraction hit, and consequently feeling it everywhere, I could relax the rest of my body and just float through it.

My choice of location and caregivers turned out to be ideal as well. I was attended by one nurse and my midwife, who simply stood back and let me be in charge of the experience, offering words of support when warranted and periodically checking the baby's heart rate with a stethoscope—but nothing more.

All in all, it was an exhilarating, empowering, incredible experience. It was exactly what I'd hoped it would be."

PLANNING FOR POSTPARTUM

Your birth plan shouldn't end with your baby's entry into the world. The minutes, hours, days, and weeks after your baby's birth are just as important for both of you.

Around the world new mothers all need the same thing—we need to be mothered so we can mother our babies. Most cultures have customs that ensure this. But in the United States today, if you don't plan for it ahead of time, you may not have the care and support you need to help you learn how to be a mother.

You and your baby's most important goals after birth should be to recover, to get acquainted, and to establish breastfeeding. To help you achieve these goals, your birth plan should include ways to develop and maintain confidence in yourself and your baby, to have support, and to stay together as much as possible.

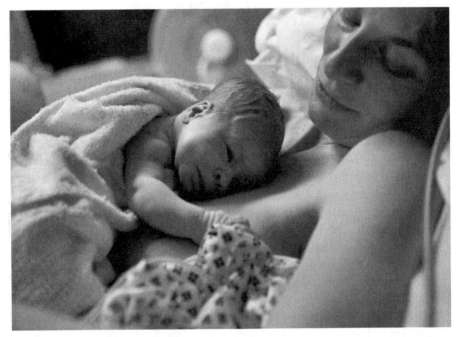

Recovering from Birth

The word *recover* means both "to regain health" and "to regain balance." You and your baby aren't sick, but you do both need to adjust physically, emotionally, and socially. Following are some strategies that may help.

In the First Days

- Make rest a top priority.
- Remember to eat and drink. Keep handy a variety of tasty, easy, nutritious snacks that you can eat with one hand.
- Make sure your support team is in place.
- Have someone hold your baby while you shower or bring your sleeping baby into the bathroom while you shower.
- Let others mother you.
- Stay active but don't get overtired.
- Eliminate nonessential work and activities.
- Talk about your birth.
- Keep your baby close.

In the First Weeks

- Ask for help with cooking, cleaning, shopping, laundry, and care of older children.
- Eat meals you made and froze before birth.
- Have takeout food during the first weeks to save your energy.
- Spend time night and day with your baby.
- Continue to limit nonessential work and activities.

Having Support

Who will be most helpful to you after your baby's birth? Your support people will be very important in the first days and weeks, so choose them carefully. They should value and support your breastfeeding and your work as a mother. They should make you feel comfortable and competent. At the very least, they should be willing to work hard. One hard-working full-time helper will do, or a number of helpers may share the load.

How to Plan for Support

- Ask your baby's grandmother to stay with you for the first week.
- Ask your partner to take vacation time or parental leave after your baby is born.
- Hire a teen to spend three hours every afternoon doing household chores.
- Interview and hire a professional postpartum doula. Unlike a baby nurse, who will only care for your baby, a postpartum

doula cares for you, helps you with breastfeeding and baby care, and does simple but important household chores, such as light cleaning, cooking, and laundry.

- Interview potential health caregivers for your baby and choose one who listens well, respects your questions, encourages and supports breastfeeding, and makes you feel comfortable and competent.

Getting Acquainted

Before your baby's birth, you may find it helpful to learn about babies from the people and resources around you, so you know generally what to expect. Your best teacher, though, will be your baby. You'll learn the most important lessons about how to be a mother simply by watching and responding to your child.

- Before birth, read the book *Your Amazing Newborn*[13] and watch the related video *Amazing Talents of the Newborn*[14]. (For more information, see Recommended Resources.)
- Before birth, spend time with other mothers and babies.
- From the moment of birth, stay close to your baby. Spend time together skin-to-skin often in the first few days.
- If you give birth at a hospital, room in with your baby.
- At home, have your baby sleep in your bedroom—in your bed, in a "sidecar" sleeper, or in a cradle, bassinet, or crib close to your bed. (See page 209 for more information on safe cosleeping.)
- Wear your baby in a sling or other soft baby carrier as you move through your day.
- Postpone guests who expect to be waited on and who distract you from your baby's needs. Welcome guests who are eager to help, freeing you and your baby to rest and get acquainted.
- Look for early infant feeding cues (see page 198) and respond to them as quickly as possible.
- Learn what comforts your baby by experimenting with a variety of infant soothing techniques, like swaddling, rocking, cuddling, listening to music, or dancing.
- Attend a La Leche League meeting, where you can nurse your baby, learn about breastfeeding, and

socialize with other mothers and babies in a relaxed and helpful atmosphere.
- Look for other mother-baby support groups at your neighborhood community center, church, or clinic.

Establishing Breastfeeding

Breastfeeding is nature's most powerful way of helping mothers recover from birth, learn mothering skills, and fall in love with their babies. It's also nature's way of ensuring that babies are well nourished, protected against disease, and allowed to develop optimally. The American Academy of Pediatrics (AAP) recommends that babies be exclusively breastfed (no water, juice, formula, other fluids, or solids) for six months and continue breastfeeding until at least one year.[15] Following are some ways you can get your breastfeeding relationship off to a good start. (For more information and advice on breastfeeding, see Chapter 12, pages 198–202, and Chapter 13, pages 211–213.)

Before Birth
- Talk to women who are breastfeeding or have breastfed babies.
- Watch babies at the breast.
- Attend a La Leche League meeting.
- Get the name of a lactation consultant.
- Read about breastfeeding in *Lamaze Parents* magazine.
- Buy a breastfeeding book like *The Ultimate Breastfeeding Book of Answers* by Jack Newman. (For more information, see Recommended Resources.)
- Remember that your body knows how to breastfeed your baby.
- Talk to your caregiver about delaying newborn testing and other routine procedures.

In the First Hours
- Keep your baby skin-to-skin with you.
- Watch for early infant feeding cues.
- Nurse your baby within the first hour after birth.

- Delay newborn tests and routine procedures until after the first breastfeeding.
- Remember that colostrum is nutrient-rich and that your baby doesn't need to eat much in the first hours and days of life.

In the First Days

- Sleep in the same room with your baby and be together as much as possible.
- Don't limit your baby's time at the breast or hold your baby off between feedings.
- Let your baby finish the first breast before offering the other.
- Learn how to tell if your baby is swallowing milk.
- Become a confident nurser by learning how to tell if your baby is getting enough milk and trusting that you will produce lots of milk.
- Learn how to position your baby for a good latch.
- Don't use bottles or pacifiers until breastfeeding is well established.
- Be patient with yourself and your baby as you both learn to breastfeed.
- If you choose to have your baby circumcised, wait at least twenty-four hours after birth and insist that he be given pain medication. Be prepared to provide extra soothing and wake your baby to breastfeed if necessary.
- If you need to be separated from your baby, pump your breasts and store your milk.
- Don't supplement your breast milk with formula unless there is a clear, compelling health reason.
- Remember that colostrum is nutrient-rich and that your baby doesn't need to eat much in the first hours and days of life.

In the First Weeks

- Remember that responding to your baby's needs does not spoil him; rather, it's the only way you can teach your baby to trust you.
- Sleep in the same room with your baby and be together as much as possible.

- Wear your baby in a sling or other soft baby carrier throughout the day.
- Nurse your baby whenever he or she shows signs of hunger (eight to twelve times every twenty-four hours).
- Learn to nurse lying down in bed so you don't need to wake fully to nurse at night.
- Remember that breastfeeding is a top priority.
- Be patient with yourself and your baby as you learn to breastfeed.
- Stay confident, even if your breastfeeding journey is bumpy.
- Call a lactation consultant, your local La Leche League leader, or the La Leche League hotline (847-519-7730) if you have breastfeeding problems or you're concerned about whether your baby is getting enough milk.
- Remember that breast milk is all the nutrition your baby needs for at least six months.

If You're Not Able to Breastfeed

Here are some tips to promote bonding and development even if you're not able to breastfeed your baby:

- Sleep in the same room with your baby and be together as much as possible.
- Wear your baby in a sling or other soft baby carrier throughout the day.
- Respond to your baby's needs before he or she cries.
- Hold your baby, make eye contact, and talk to your baby during feedings.
- Hold, look at, and talk to your baby even when you're not feeding.

READY FOR THE JOURNEY

You've made your plans. You've folded and refolded all the tiny undershirts. You've organized your baby's layette a dozen times. The days may drag as you await your baby's arrival. But that special day will indeed arrive—and it's coming soon.

Relax and savor the last days of your pregnancy. Take a long walk. Enjoy a special food you crave. Rest and pamper yourself. Have your hair trimmed or get a manicure. Window shop. Water your plants. Have a leisurely cup of tea with a friend. Lie down with a book and drift into a nap. Have a candlelight dinner with your partner and ignore the phone.

Even if you're at your job until labor begins, mental preparation can help you feel rested, calm, and well equipped. Place a flower at your workstation. Eat a tasty, healthy snack. Take a stroll on your lunch break. Spend a few minutes using relaxation techniques at your desk.

When labor finally starts, you'll be rested, relaxed, and ready for the journey. The passage from pregnancy to motherhood is the most exciting, life-changing journey you'll ever take.

Chapter 11

COMMUNICATION
AND NEGOTIATION

Good plans shape good decisions.
That's why good planning helps to
make elusive dreams come true.
—Lester Bittel

Making important decisions is always challenging. Making a
decision when pregnancy or labor isn't going as you'd hoped
or making a decision that requires your caregiver to practice
differently than usual can be especially hard.

If you want a normal birth, chances are at some point
during pregnancy, labor, or postpartum you'll find yourself
discussing and negotiating your care with a powerful, perhaps
intimidating healthcare system. Even if you've chosen your
caregiver and birth site carefully, you'll still face the reality
that normal birth isn't the norm in the United States.

To make real-life decisions that you believe are best for
you and *your baby* (as opposed to hypothetical decisions that
are statistically best for mothers and babies collectively), you
need complete, accurate, up-to-date information. You need
confidence in your knowledge, your body, and your rights. You
need to be aware of the potential obstacles to normal birth so
you're not caught by surprise. And of course, you need to be
able to communicate clearly, honestly, and respectfully.

It's hard to be nonconformist, especially when you're in
unfamiliar territory and feeling vulnerable. We hope this chapter
will make your job a little easier by giving you some practical
strategies for communicating and negotiating with the healthcare
system. We also hope the stories on the following pages,
which show informed decision making in action, will
encourage and inspire you.

STRATEGIES

Be Alert

Getting caught off-guard can put you at an emotional and practical disadvantage. To avoid unpleasant surprises, be aware of the following issues that tend to pop up around pregnancy and birth. Many caregivers and hospitals in the U.S.:

• assume all expectant mothers want a full range of prenatal tests;
• induce labor before forty-two weeks, sometimes as early as thirty-seven weeks;
• speed up labor when they think it's taking too long;
• routinely use continuous electronic fetal monitoring and intravenous fluids;
• separate mothers and babies after birth;
• restrict movement and position during labor;
• support elective cesarean surgery;
• do cesareans when they think labor has gone on too long;
• discourage vaginal birth after a cesarean (VBAC).

You should also be prepared for pressure to go along with the options presented to you. Your caregiver or hospital may use "safety" to persuade you, suggesting risks you incur if you don't go with the program. Or you may be promised less pain or a shorter labor.

Remember that the specific risk for you and your baby—unique individuals in unique circumstances—is different from the statistical risk for all mothers and babies collectively. Remember, too, that usually the easier, healthier way to give birth is with nature in the driver's seat. Make your decisions calmly and deliberately, according to best evidence and careful consideration of your situation and your values, not by reacting emotionally.

Be Informed

You probably already know a great deal about normal birth from reading this book, talking to others, taking classes, and doing research of your own. If an unfamiliar issue arises, you can find out more about it. It's always a good idea to have a complete understanding of the issue at hand before making a decision.

You can quickly and easily find excellent, evidence-based, up-to-date information about pregnancy, birth, and baby care by checking *Effective Care in Pregnancy and Childbirth: A Synopsis* in Appendix A of this book. (See page 229.) Many other trustworthy books and videos are listed in Recommended Resources (page 289). If online research is more your style, visit the following informative, user-friendly websites.

- http://www.maternitywise.org (Maternity Center Association)
- http://www.normalbirth.lamaze.org (Lamaze Institute for Normal Birth)
- http://www.acnm.org (American College of Nurse-Midwives)
- http://www.motherfriendly.org (Coalition for Improving Maternity Services)
- http://www.lalecheleague.com (La Leche League International)

Be Confident

Be confident in the knowledge you've worked so hard to acquire. If you don't feel confident in your knowledge, learn more until you do.

Be confident in your body and your baby. We hope this book has given you all the reasons you need to trust nature's plan for pregnancy and birth, as well as your ability to carry out that plan.

Be confident that no one cares more about your well-being and your baby's well-being than you do, and no one is better qualified to make decisions about you and your baby. Furthermore, it's your right and responsibility to make such decisions. Unless you're incapacitated or facing an emergency that puts your life or your baby's life in immediate peril, you have the right to decline practices that you feel aren't in your best interest.

Be a Good Communicator

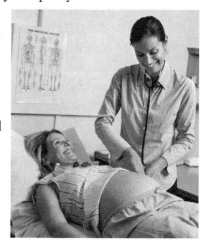

When you're faced with a choice about your care in pregnancy or birth, it's critical to ask questions. Regardless of your circumstances, the following tips can encourage dialogue, help you get the information you need, and promote negotiation and understanding.

- Ask for more information about what's being recommended or offered. For example, ask, "Could you tell me more about this?" Or say, "I'd like a better understanding of why you recommend this for me."
- Inquire about alternatives. For example, ask, "Are there other things I could do?" Or ask, "What other options are there?" If you've heard of an alternative, ask about that.
- Ask, "What will happen if I wait?"
- Ask, "What are the risks of doing nothing?"
- Consider the response you get in the context of what you already know. Don't be afraid to point out what you know or mention that your knowledge differs from what you're now hearing.
- Try not to put your caregiver or hospital staff on the defensive. Use "I" statements to keep the focus on you and avoid pointing fingers. Remember that this is a conversation, not a debate. You don't need to change anyone else's beliefs; you're simply gathering information and making a personal choice.

STORIES

Margaret

I didn't think I wanted a routine sonogram with my second baby, but at the last minute I thought, "Why not?" So I went ahead with it.

I was shocked when my midwife called and told me the sonogram showed "something strange in part of the brain." I asked her what that meant, and she said she didn't know. She encouraged me to talk directly to the doctor who read the sonogram.

I called several times, and finally he returned my call. He said he'd only seen it once before, and that baby was fine. He said one option was to have a more sophisticated sonogram to get a better look. I asked what further information that would give. He said he didn't know. I asked what would happen if I did nothing, and he said that it would probably make no difference.

I was particularly concerned that if there were something seriously wrong with my baby, it might not be wise to give birth in the birth center I was planning to use. I asked about that. I also wanted to know if additional information would change the course of my pregnancy, since I planned to have my baby no matter what.

The doctor reassured me that what he saw was probably "clinically insignificant" and that it didn't have implications for where I gave birth or the course of my pregnancy. I told him that based on our discussion, I wouldn't have more testing.

He responded, "I think you are very wise."

Margaret's story is a good example of a thoughtful discussion in which both parties communicate honestly and openly. Margaret communicated her concerns clearly, and her doctor shared honestly what could be learned from additional testing without trying to sway her decision. Based on this discussion, Margaret was able to make an informed choice. Her decision was actually an informed refusal to do additional testing.

Robin

I had my first three babies in Haiti. I was shocked when I arrived at the hospital for the birth of my fourth baby (in the U. S.) and learned I was expected to stay in bed. I asked why. The nurse said that the hospital policy was that all laboring women had to stay in bed.

I said, "I've had three babies. I know how to labor. I walk and rock and moan. And I can't do that in bed." The nurse tried to convince me that it was important to be in bed.

I couldn't listen to her. I got out of bed, went out the door, and walked up and down the halls, moaning with the contractions. The nurse called my doctor, but I didn't care.

When he arrived, I told him, "I know how to be in labor." He shrugged his shoulders, and they let me keep walking.

When I felt the urge to push, I let the nurse know, went back to my room, and pushed my baby out.

Robin's first three births made her very confident that she knew just what she needed to do in labor. She wasn't the least bit intimidated by the hospital environment. Her determination was difficult for the hospital staff to fight. And her self-assurance was probably contagious!

Mary

I arrived at the birth center in hard labor at 7:00 A.M. I was already seven centimeters dilated. My midwife asked if I wanted her to break my water. I asked why.

My midwife said, "The baby's head is right there. If I break your water, you will have your baby very quickly. Otherwise, it will probably be an hour or so."

My labor was moving just about as fast as I could handle. A quicker labor was tempting, but I reminded myself that a fast labor isn't as important as being able to work with labor—which I was just barely able to do.

I told her I didn't want her to break my water, that I was okay with labor taking a bit longer. I went into the tub, stayed there about an hour, then got out and had my baby.

Even in hard labor, Mary was focused enough to ask the right question: Why? She could then figure out whether the option being offered made sense for her. She decided that a faster birth wasn't a benefit for her. She communicated her wishes effectively to her midwife, who listened to her.

Linda

I had a cesarean for my first birth. I labored on a stretcher in a hallway for six hours because there were no beds available in the labor suite. I was unable to move. In retrospect it's not surprising that I made no progress, and that my doctor then convinced me and my husband that I needed a cesarean.

With my second baby I found a doctor who told me I could try for a VBAC. I also attended Lamaze classes, and when we discussed birth plans and communicating with our doctors, my childbirth educator encouraged me to start asking questions.

So I did. My doctor kept insisting I could have a trial of labor, but as my due date came closer he began to talk about the advantages of another cesarean. I asked him how many of his patients actually gave birth vaginally after a cesarean.

He evaded the question and then talked at length about the risks of VBAC.

My husband and I decided it was clear he wasn't supporting our plan for a trial of labor. We discovered later from a nurse at the hospital that he had never attended a VBAC.

I asked my childbirth educator to recommend a doctor who supported VBACs. Our insurance wouldn't pay for the new doctor, but a normal birth was important enough to us that we were willing to pay ourselves.

We changed doctors at thirty-seven weeks. Our families weren't supportive. They were sure our doctor was protecting us from ourselves and that it was safer to have another cesarean. But we were sure of our decision.

I gave birth to a nine-and-a-half-pound baby girl after four hours of labor. It was an incredible experience. We're so glad we asked questions, got the information we needed, and made the decision to change doctors.

Linda's questioning and her increasing awareness of her doctor's mixed messages compelled her to consider other options. It was hard to change doctors late in her pregnancy, and the pressure from family made it even harder. But Linda and her husband were well informed, and they knew what they wanted.

Jen

I developed gestational diabetes, and at thirty-seven weeks my doctor started talking about inducing if I didn't go into labor in the next week or so. I asked why, and she told me that she always worried about being late with gestational diabetes.

I looked at the information in The Cochrane Library *and talked to my aunt, who's a childbirth educator. I knew my baby wasn't in danger, and neither was I.*

But I felt so pressured by my doctor. I didn't want a medical induction. I wanted to go into labor naturally. I asked her what would happen if we just waited. She told me that my baby might be too big if we waited until my due date, and then I would need a cesarean.

*Again, I researched and found this wasn't true. I asked
my doula if she had ideas for encouraging labor to start
naturally. At her suggestion, over the next two weeks I did
visualization and went twice a week for acupuncture.*

*At thirty-nine weeks I went into labor on my own.
I arrived at the hospital eight centimeters dilated after
three hours of labor. And my baby was seven pounds!*

Jen's story is a common one. Many women are tempted by
induction—the last weeks of pregnancy are hard, and it's
natural to want to hold one's baby at last. And in Jen's case,
"safety" was offered as another reason for induction. But Jen
knew that an unnecessary induction could make her labor
more difficult and start a cascade of interventions. She
wanted to increase her chances of having a normal birth.
So she learned more about both gestational diabetes and
induction, and as a result, she stopped worrying about
nonexistent risks. She also found alternatives that helped her
body go into labor naturally.

Sheila

*A week before my due date, early in the morning, my water
broke. When I called my midwife, she reassured me and said
I should expect contractions to start soon.*

*Twelve hours later she called back to ask what was
happening. Nothing. She wanted us to come to the hospital,
to get started on antibiotics, to get some sleep. If there were
still no contractions in the morning, she'd induce labor.*

*We didn't want to go to the hospital yet, or to be induced.
We asked what the alternatives were and what would happen
if we waited awhile.*

*Our midwife made it clear that although she believed
labor would start in the next twelve hours if we stayed at
home, she was mandated to follow hospital protocol, which
was admission to the hospital and antibiotics after twelve
hours from rupture of membranes.*

*I would've just gone to the hospital, but my husband
reminded me of the cascade of interventions. We told the
midwife we wanted to stay home, and if contractions hadn't*

*started by morning (twenty-four hours after my water broke),
we'd come to the hospital then.*

*The midwife agreed, but said she'd have to document our
refusal to come to the hospital at twelve hours. We were fine
with that.*

*At 3:00 A.M. contractions started. We arrived at the
hospital in active labor at 11:00 A.M. But the pressure of
waiting for labor to begin had taken its toll; I was exhausted
when labor got intense. Still, I'm glad we did what we did.
I did get antibiotics but avoided induction.*

*For our second baby, I chose a midwifery practice in a
birth center that had less restrictive policies in hopes that
my midwives wouldn't feel pressured and pass that pressure
on to me.*

Sheila's story is an example of hospital policy dictating
caregiver practice. Sheila and her midwife were both in a
bind. Based on best evidence, there was no reason to hurry
labor just yet. Their compromise was to note Sheila's refusal
on her chart. But the decision to stay at home didn't alleviate
the pressure that Sheila felt to have labor start. Ultimately,
labor did start on its own—and despite Sheila's exhaustion,
she gave birth normally to a healthy baby girl.

Michelle

*I started having contractions about 6:00 P.M., and at 7:30
my mother insisted I call my doctor. I refused, but she was
insistent. She said she knew all the signs and that I was
moving quickly.*

*She was right. When we arrived at the hospital at 8:15,
I was nine centimeters dilated. By the time I got to my room,
the nurse said to go ahead and push if I felt like it.*

*I didn't really, but I tried. Then I hung out and waited
about an hour until I felt the urge. I was full of energy, but
my baby just wasn't moving down. My doula and mother and
husband encouraged me and helped me into lots of different
positions. My baby was doing fine.*

*At midnight—after almost four hours of pushing—I was
still at it. I still had energy, and my baby was still doing fine.
But my team was discouraged, and I was needing a pep talk.*

My doctor came in, and I asked what was happening. She said she didn't think I could push the baby out. I asked what would happen if we waited, since my baby and I were okay. Her answer? "You can push for another hour or two, but it won't make any difference. That baby isn't going anywhere. You're going to have a cesarean now or later."

I was terribly disappointed, but when she said that all my confidence went. I had no energy to keep going.

All Michelle needed to keep going was a boost of confidence. And since both she and her baby were doing well, it made sense to keep trying a bit longer. She asked the right questions, but was understandably vulnerable when her doctor told her that her hard work was futile. She'll never know if another hour would've made a difference. She now wishes she had insisted on pushing longer, and with her next baby she plans to use a midwife who won't give up on her so easily.

YOUR JOURNEY

The path of your pregnancy, labor, birth, and postpartum will be uniquely yours. Along the way you may encounter bumps that require interventions you hadn't anticipated or bumps that require you to steadfastly refuse interventions.

Only you can figure out what's best for you. You'll make good decisions if you have full, accurate information, if you communicate honestly and openly with your caregiver, and if you have confidence in yourself.

Chapter 12

GREETING
YOUR NEWBORN

*A child is born, and for a moment the
wheeling planets seem to stop in their tracks,
as past, present and future meet.*
—Sheila Kitzinger

This chapter describes the events that should occur in the
hours after giving birth as well as events that may occur
in some birth settings. It also discusses your newborn's
appearance, abilities, and behavior and expands on the
importance of breastfeeding. Greeting your newborn should
be a time to cherish. Prepare to protect it by reading the
following sections carefully, asking questions about your
birth site's policies and protocol, and making your wishes
known *before* you give birth.

BABYMOON:
THE MAGICAL TIME
FOLLOWING BIRTH

Nothing can describe the moments
when you first gaze at your newborn's
face and the following hours when
you marvel at everything she does.
Anthropologist Sheila Kitzinger
calls this brief, precious period the
"babymoon" and reminds parents that
it's something more than a sequel to
delivery.[1] The babymoon is another
part of the beautiful, unique dance
between mother and child. These first

hours establish the foundation of your future together, allowing love, trust, and understanding to grow.

During the babymoon, a mother and her newborn need time that's unhurried by the clock. But depending on where the birth occurs, getting plenty of uninterrupted time may prove difficult. If you give birth in a hospital, standard protocol is designed to make every procedure efficient, safe, and identical for every patient—and this usually requires following a strict timetable. Your baby's umbilical cord may be clamped and cut within a minute or two after birth. You may be hurried to birth your placenta, rather than birthing it at your own pace. The staff may want to examine your baby in a warming bed, put medicine in her eyes, and dress her in a warmed gown and blanket. They may wish to further observe and treat your baby in the nursery.

If you give birth at home or in a birth center, your midwife knows that there's no reason to separate you and your baby during the first few hours. Someone can assess your baby's health without removing her from your arms (the safest place for your baby to be). Your baby's umbilical cord doesn't need to be cut immediately, and you don't need to birth your placenta right away. Your midwife understands the importance of protecting the hours after birth, when you should have the quiet privacy to "learn" your baby while you're both alert, to hear her sounds and smell her newborn odors, to stretch out her little legs for a first diaper change, to gaze and to fall in love.

The hours after birth can be just as intense as those during labor, and the initial moments can be a real shock. You may find yourself holding your newborn and wondering, "Is this really happening to me?" Your body is exhausted from the hard work it's done. The rush of adrenalin during your final pushes may have left you trembling and your teeth chattering. These physical reactions may be accompanied by an emotional high unlike any other. You may weep or laugh uncontrollably. A blanket and a pair of socks will help control the trembling and chattering teeth—and undisturbed, uninterrupted time with your newborn will help focus your emotions.

During these first few hours, no one needs to show you how to bond with your baby. You both simply need the privacy, peace, patience, and confidence to do what your bodies, hearts, and minds already know how to do. If you're giving birth in a hospital, the staff's job is to create a quiet, intimate environment for you and your baby's first hours together, even if it's handling twenty other births at the same time. It's your job to diligently prepare for the event and discuss your wishes with caregivers and staff until you're satisfied with their responses and you're certain everyone understands your expectations for birth and beyond.

Some hospital midwives encourage their clients to write to hospital administrators about any grievances they have with outdated policies that separate them from their healthy babies. Hospital regulations get changed and brought up to date only after complaints and requests are repeatedly made.

Navajo midwife Ursula Knoki-Wilson talks about the sacred moments after a baby's birth at her clinic. "It's a time of listening, of mutual respect, of dignity, and harmony. The mother and father shake the baby's hand at birth, honoring this little one as a separate individual. And then they formally name the baby: 'Hello, my baby, (Navajo name). You come into my hands riding on a beautiful white (or other color) horse.'"[2] The unhurried hours after the baby's birth are important ceremonial ones that build strong bonds between baby and parents.

THE IMPORTANCE OF BONDING

In the late 1960s two pediatricians, Marshall Klaus and John Kennell, noticed that hospital routines denied mothers and babies the opportunity to get to know each other after birth. Their subsequent research revealed a "sensitive period" in the first hours after birth and showed the importance of the intense connection (bonding) of mother and baby during that time. Their research demonstrated that spending this brief time together resulted in healthier children and stronger attachments between the babies and mothers.[3] It became the impetus for changing hospital routines to give mothers undisturbed time with their newborns.

The following sections describe skin-to-skin contact and rooming in—two practices that not only facilitate bonding, but also help both mother and baby in amazing ways during the first hours and days after birth.

Skin-to-Skin: The Best Place to Be

Just as the best place for your baby to grow from conception was in your womb, the best place for him right after birth is on your skin, not in a warmer or another person's arms. This skin-to-skin contact is also called "kangaroo care," because the natural warmth, protection, and nutrition a mother's body offers her newborn is like the safe haven a baby kangaroo enjoys in its mother's pouch. Ina May Gaskin and her team of midwives at the Farm Midwifery Center designed their postpartum routines around this skin-to-skin time. They believe that mother and baby "are doing something more important than just lying together. They are falling in love."[4]

After you give birth, your deflated abdomen becomes a nest of loose skin for your baby. While in the nest, the skin-to-skin contact promotes the gentle, natural regulation of your baby's heart rate and body temperature. It also helps him establish regular breathing patterns and sustain high, stable blood sugar levels. Exposure to the natural bacteria on your skin during the first hours reduces his risk of illness from germs in the environment. Newborns who have skin-to-skin contact with their mothers cry very little, if at all—compare this reaction to the often upset babies who are examined and warmed in a warmer across the room or in the hospital nursery. It makes sense that babies respond well to touch. For forty weeks, a baby is in constant contact with his mother's body.

Skin-to skin contact can facilitate breastfeeding. Researchers in Sweden have discovered that when a newborn is placed on his mother's abdomen, in time he can make his way to his mother's breast and actually latch on by himself.[5] Baby is helped along by the familiar smell of amniotic fluid on his hands, the smell and warmth of his mother's skin, the sound of her voice, and the "target" of her darkened nipple.

Skin-to-skin contact can also benefit you by keeping oxytocin levels high. After giving birth, your uterus is the size of a grapefruit. In the hours and days that follow, contractions are needed to help shrink it to its normal pear size. Oxytocin levels are very high as your baby moves through your birth canal and remain high as you and your newborn first touch each other, stare into each other's eyes, and breastfeed together. The high levels of oxytocin keep your uterus contracted to reduce bleeding. Oxytocin is also partly responsible for the "falling in love" feeling you have when you first meet your newborn. Oxytocin helps you feel calm and responsive. In the days following birth, oxytocin helps ward off postpartum depression, continues to keep your uterus contracted, and speeds healing.

While against your skin, your baby's hand and head movements stimulate the release of additional oxytocin and endorphins, increasing milk production and keeping you and your baby calm and relaxed.[6] Endorphins have been called nature's narcotic. Research shows that when our bodies work hard, endorphin levels rise, especially when we feel secure, warm, and loved. Endorphins do more than block pain reception: in the initial moments after giving birth, endorphins help accelerate a mother's ability to bond with her baby. Endorphin levels are especially high within twenty minutes after the birth, and they're strongly present in her breast milk.

For all its physical and emotional benefits, skin-to-skin contact should be a carefully protected routine. During this intimate time, mothers become acutely aware of their newborn's needs—and who else is touching the baby and what's being done to him. Neither mother nor newborn misses a beat in the first hours when left together, and others should trust them to follow each other's lead. Baby and mother will know when it's time for a feeding, when it's time for comforting, when it's time for exploring.

To make sure you and your baby are given time for skin-to-skin contact,

Kate found out hours after her daughter's birth that a staff member had drawn blood from the baby's foot in the hospital's nursery without her or her husband's consent. "She was a big baby—almost ten pounds—and she was healthy. They took her to the nursery while they finished up with me. I guess it was routine—they thought there was a chance my big baby might be diabetic. Later, I hated discovering that little prick hole in her heel, not knowing what her reaction might have been, or even how they did it." When a newborn stays with her mother, little goes undetected in the first hours after birth.

request that he's put on your bare abdomen or chest right after birth, with a warmed receiving blanket laid over you both and a hat on his damp head to help keep the warmth in. Also request that any examination of him is done while he's in your arms. Nothing should interrupt your baby's assurance that your body is a safe haven.

Rooming In: Keeping Baby and Mother Together

Before the twentieth century, when births occurred at home, mothers and babies stayed in the same room during the first days after birth. When births moved to hospitals, the medical community believed that mothers needed to rest alone and that babies were safer when kept in nurseries. As a result, mothers saw their babies only periodically during the day for feedings, following a strict schedule set by the hospital staff.

If you give birth in a hospital, protocol may lead staff to suggest that you let them care for your baby in the nursery so you can sleep better. Make no mistake—giving birth is hard work, and rest and sleep are important in the first days. Without rest, a mother's exhaustion may lead to sickness, sadness, or feeling overwhelmed. Her tired, stressed-out behavior may lead to a cranky baby, who picks up on her mother's signals. To be the calm, rested caregiver your baby needs, it's important that you sleep and rest, but that is actually easier in close physical contact with your baby. Studies show that mothers whose babies stay in nurseries don't necessarily sleep more or any better. In fact, mothers and babies who stay together without any separation rest better.[7] You may sleep more peacefully knowing that your baby is next to you. You're there to make sure she stays warm, and you can immediately respond to her cries. During breastfeeding, high levels of prolactin and oxytocin actually help you relax and sometimes even doze off during feedings.

Rabbi Harold Kushner talks about a woman giving birth as bringing a new living soul into the world, perhaps the most creative thing anyone could do. "Just as nurturing a child within her for nine months draws on the mother's physical resources, giving that child a soul draws on her spiritual resources. It would make sense for a new mother, despite all that a newborn infant demands of her, to take time to replenish her soul in the weeks after the birth."[8] Finding time to rest and be replenished (that is, to be repaired, refilled, restored) with a newborn is an important habit to form during the first hours after birth and beyond.

Rooming in allows baby and mother to rehearse the cues and responses that help with two important developments: The mother can learn her baby's cues and needs more quickly, which means the baby can trust that her messages will get responses. This means that breastfeeding gets off to a better start, too. When your newborn awakens hungry with you holding her or just a step away, she sends signals that you've learned to recognize, and you put her to the breast well before she cries.

"It makes sense that the more time two people spend together, the sooner they get to know each other," says nurse and Lamaze childbirth educator Jeannette Crenshaw,[9] who adds that babies who room in with their mothers gain more weight per day,[10] are less likely to be become jaundiced (have yellowish skin as the liver catches up to break down red blood cells),[11] and sleep more peacefully.[12] Studies show that mothers who room in with their babies for longer periods of time—including during the night—score higher on tests that measure the strength of attachment to their babies.[13]

One of Anne's fondest memories of her daughter's home birth was the pediatrician's visit. "She was born before dawn broke, and it was sunset when the doctor arrived and came upstairs to our bedroom to check her out. She and I hadn't left the warmth of that bedroom all day, we were so content. Jenny was sleeping on my stomach, her head turned toward him, her little mouth barely opened in a relaxed O. He was Welsh and stopped midway across our very softly lit room and whispered, 'Oh, father! Get a photo of this wee baby before I take a look.' We have that picture up on our wall, of Jenny sleeping peacefully on me that first night with us. She never left that spot all the time he quietly examined her and then said goodnight to us."

A Few Final Words on Bonding

Because research shows that being together is best for mother and baby, more hospitals need to protect and promote kangaroo care and rooming in. If you plan to give birth in a hospital, make sure you ask for the time and opportunity to get to know your baby—uninterrupted and undisturbed. But also remember that forming a strong attachment to your baby is not something done only during the first few hours and days of your baby's life. Bonding is a lifetime process.

PROCEDURES AFTER BIRTH

Cutting the Umbilical Cord

The umbilical cord is a tough, flexible rope of blood vessels that connects your baby to your womb and works with the placenta to nourish him. Considering the amount of tumbling and turning a baby does in the womb, it's not surprising that the cord can end up looped around the neck. Most often it's not a cause for alarm. The birth attendant gently slips the cord over the baby's head during the birth.

At birth, the cord protrudes from your baby's navel, often pulsating for many minutes after the birth. It continues to provide him oxygen and nourishment and ease his transition to the outside world. Although many doctors clamp and cut the cord within a minute or two after birth, most research shows that the procedure isn't an urgent one.[14] There's no agreement within the medical community on how soon it should happen or how long it can be delayed. However, delaying the procedure ensures that you and your baby have some uninterrupted time to get to know each other—as long as your baby is still connected to you, no one can separate you! Delaying the procedure also gives your baby the chance to adjust to his new surroundings more calmly.

Banking Cord Blood

Umbilical cord blood contains stem cells that may be able to treat many diseases. Stem cells divide to create red and white blood cells and platelets. They're the "building blocks" of the blood, the immune system, and body tissues.

While the potential curative use of stem cells is promising, the development of stem cell research and cord blood banking is still in the early stages.

There are private and public companies that offer cord blood banking. For a fee that can range from several hundreds to thousands of dollars (depending on the company), parents can have their baby's cord blood frozen and stored, making stem cells available should the child develop a disease that these cells may be able to treat. Parents can also donate their baby's cord blood for research or for treatment. However, parents should know there's absolutely no guarantee that a cord blood transplant will offer appropriate treatment or that it'll provide a cure. There's also no guarantee that a company can successfully store the cells until they're needed—or that it'll stay in business.

The American Academy of Pediatrics (AAP) believes that because there's a lack of evidence that an individual child would ever need stored umbilical cord blood, it's difficult to recommend that parents store their children's cord blood for future use. The AAP also expresses concern that families are especially vulnerable to emotional marketing at the time of birth.[15]

If you do decide to store your baby's cord blood, it's important that you don't let the collection procedure (which is painless) prevent you from keeping your baby skin-to-skin in the first minutes after birth.

Birthing the Placenta

Your placenta grew with your baby in the womb from the cells of the fertilized egg. Through the umbilical cord, it nourished, maintained, and protected your baby throughout your pregnancy. The placenta is also called the afterbirth; however, birthing the placenta is an important part of the process of birth. Your uterus continues to contract after your baby's born, gently loosening and separating the placenta from the uterine wall. Keeping your baby skin-to-skin exerts gentle pressure on your uterus, and your baby's movements on your chest stimulate your body to release increasing amounts of oxytocin. This is nature's way of encouraging the placenta to separate and deliver.

How and when you birth your placenta depends on where the birth occurs. Many hospitals set a specific time limit on when you should birth the placenta (usually within five minutes of your baby's birth). Hospital staff often hurry the birth of the placenta by tugging on the umbilical cord or by applying strong pressure to the top of your abdomen, and many doctors give intravenous (IV) Pitocin to stimulate the uterus to stay contracted and deliver the placenta quickly. All these practices are potentially harmful.

Other caregivers let you birth the placenta on your own and at your own pace. You're not rushed in any way. Instead, you spend the first minutes after the birth concentrating on your baby, holding and touching her as you get to know each other. Later on, your midwife or birth attendant might help you sit up or squat so gravity can help bring down the placenta. You might push it out, just as you pushed your baby out. Holding and nursing your baby encourages the uterus to contract and expel the placenta. This less aggressive process takes about twenty minutes but may quite safely take longer—and you will have your baby in your arms the entire time.

The placenta is an amazing, life-giving organ that sometimes gets ignored in the rush of birth. Some women have no desire to see it. But some do. These women describe the placenta as beautiful—its network of blood vessels looking like a tree of life.

In his book *Childbirth without Fear*, Grantly Dick-Read said that in the past not many of his patients wanted to see the placenta. "Today, nearly every mother who watches her baby born asks me to show her the placenta. This I do, and I point out the bag in which the infant, now lying peacefully in her arms, developed and became a perfect little human being."[16]

More and more women attach symbolism to the placenta, recognizing it as an important life source for their babies. Many cultures around the world observe rituals that honor the placenta: a ceremonial planting of it in ancestral land (Maori); special preparation and use of its potential "life-source" power in certain medicines (Chinese); washing, wrapping, and burying it as a "sibling" of the newborn (Malaysian). Many women request to keep the placenta, then later plant it with a tree or shrub in honor of the newborn. If you give birth in a hospital, its policy may be to use the placenta for skin grafts and treatment of burn victims, or it may simply discard or incinerate the placenta.

Whatever you'd like done with your placenta, make the decision before birth and make your wishes known to everyone attending your birth. This way, its fate won't be decided without your input during the exciting moments when everyone's busy meeting your newborn.

Checking the Apgar Score and Birth Weight and Length

At one minute and again at five minutes after birth, your midwife, a nurse, or another birth attendant will check your baby's breathing, heart rate, skin color, muscle tone, and reflexes. This procedure is called the Apgar score after Virginia Apgar, the anesthesiologist who first suggested compiling a score to assess a newborn's overall condition. The birth attendant observes the baby and gives points for how well the baby's adjusting to life outside the womb. The higher the score, the better the baby's adjustment.

These simple observations are visual only and are subjective. There's no reason why your baby needs to be taken from you while being observed. The birth attendant can check your baby quietly and as efficiently as possible—while he's still in your arms or on your chest.

Your baby's weight and length don't need to be measured immediately after birth. These assessments can wait until you and your baby have had some uninterrupted time together.

Screenings and Other Routine Procedures

Healthcare officials, state health agencies, researchers, and parents will likely never agree on what tests should or should not be given to a newborn. Individual states may offer exemptions to routine procedures for medical, religious, or philosophical reasons.

Before your baby's birth, learn all you can about the following tests and procedures. Contact a local hospital or your state's public health department to find out what other tests and procedures your state mandates.

Vitamin K

Vitamin K helps the blood clot. Although babies are born with extremely low levels of it, colostrum (the mother's first breast milk) is rich in vitamin K. Although giving a newborn vitamin K (either orally or by injection) is mandatory in many states, its necessity—and risk—is controversial. Some medical reports claim that the mandatory administration of vitamin K may not be based on sound science.[17] Some studies recommend that hospitals change their policies so only newborns at risk of blood clotting problems get vitamin K. These are babies who were born prematurely or by cesarean section, whose mothers' diets were low in vitamin K during pregnancy, or whose mothers took drugs or antibiotics during pregnancy.

Administering vitamin K exemplifies how medical science can create a problem that it must solve with yet another intervention. After World War II, American research determined that formula was superior to breast milk, and consequently more babies were formula-fed than breastfed. However, formula doesn't contain the vitamin K that's naturally present in breast milk, so the mandates to administer vitamin K to newborns arose to remedy this problem.

A more natural, reasonable approach to providing newborns with vitamin K is to encourage mothers to eat adequate amounts of foods with vitamin K (such as leafy green vegetables) during pregnancy and after birth so their breast milk contains it. Breastfeeding your baby should give him enough vitamin K naturally if you're getting enough of the vitamin yourself, and, even more importantly, if you make sure that he receives plenty of hind milk (the last milk of each feeding) when he breastfeeds.

Well before your baby's birth, find out your state's laws about administering vitamin K to newborns. Make an informed decision about vitamin K and communicate your wishes to your birth attendants. If you can't opt out of the shot or oral dosage, ask that the treatment be delayed for at least an hour or until your baby has breastfed and adjusted to the surroundings.

Eye Drops or Ointment

To prevent gonorrhea and other infections from attacking a newborn's vision, many states mandate hospitals to administer antibiotic eye drops or ointment in the eyes of all infants, even if they have not been exposed to gonorrhea or other sexually transmitted diseases. These drops are gentler than they were in the past (none of them, however, catches all sexually transmitted diseases), but they still can irritate many babies' eyes. Although this procedure may be mandatory, parents can opt out of it. Check your state's mandates on eye treatment. If you can't opt out of it, delay the procedure for an hour or at least until after your baby has breastfed and adjusted to the surroundings. After all, he can't see when his eyes are covered in medicine.

Phenylketonuria Screening

Phenylketonuria (PKU) screening is a blood test that looks for a very rare problem with your baby's metabolism. Babies with PKU don't have the enzyme to process the proteins they eat, leading to possible mental and physical problems. Treatment is usually dietary.

In most states, the screening is mandatory within two to six days after birth, once your baby has eaten and digestion is functioning. Oftentimes, a baby's heel is pricked to get the blood sample, a painful procedure. Breastfeeding during any painful procedure will decrease your baby's perception of pain dramatically.[18]

Glucose Screening

Hospitals give a glucose screening (blood sugar test) to babies who are under five pounds or over nine pounds at birth, or if mother is diabetic. These babies are at risk for developing low blood sugar in the first hours of life. Babies who show signs of low blood sugar (trembling or shaking) are also tested. The best way to prevent low blood sugar in your baby is to nurse him soon and often. And if your baby does indeed develop low blood sugar, breastfeeding is the best medicine.[19]

Hepatitis B Vaccination

Hepatitis B is a serious disease caused by a virus that attacks the liver. It is a sexually transmitted disease, and can also be transmitted by blood. If you have active hepatitis or are a chronic carrier, your baby will be given the hepatitis B vaccine shortly after birth. The vaccine is mandatory for all newborns in many hospitals. The AAP recommends that infants receive a first dose either in the first days after birth, or at one month. Learn about the benefits and risks of the hepatitis B vaccine before your baby is born. Make sure the hospital staff knows your wishes about the vaccination.

Vaccinations

Healthcare providers, state health agencies, researchers, and parents will likely never agree on what vaccines a child should receive. And experts don't seem to agree on the number of vaccinations, when they should be given, and how the vaccines should be combined in a given injection. Before your baby is two years old, he may receive vaccinations for diphtheria, tetanus, pertussis (whooping cough), influenza, polio, measles, mumps, rubella, pneumococcal conjugate, and chicken pox. Some babies react to a vaccination with a fever, vomiting, or lethargy. It's worth learning about each vaccine beforehand so you can discuss its effectiveness and necessity with your baby's caregiver more knowledgeably. Some states offer exemptions to routine vaccinations for medical, religious, or philosophical reasons. Keep in mind that the first and most important "vaccine" your baby should receive is your breast milk. The immunities, antibodies, and countless other protections will benefit your baby for as long as you breastfeed him.

Deciding about Circumcision

One of the least agreed-upon procedures in the American medical community is circumcision. This procedure involves cutting off the foreskin from the tip of the penis. Once a routine procedure, questions about the necessity of circumcision have risen in the past few decades. A longtime belief that supports circumcision is its potential medical benefits, like its ability to lower the risk of urinary tract infections, penile cancer, and some sexually transmitted diseases. The evidence, however, indicates that circumcised boys are only slightly more protected from these problems than intact (uncircumcised) boys and that other factors (like diet and behavior) better determine risk. Other reasons for circumcision are religious beliefs, social customs (for example, circumcision makes boys look like their fathers), and cultural beliefs (for example, the mistaken belief that circumcision makes hygiene easier). Until the 1970s, circumcision was so routine in hospitals that parents often weren't informed before their babies had the surgery.

> "I'm glad our first baby was a girl," Shawna recalls. "We hadn't really worked out the issues around whether to circumcise. Had we consented to what the hospital wanted to do, we would have said yes at the time." The couple's son was born two years later, and after finding out more information about the procedure, they decided against circumcision. "Our son's grandfather was not circumcised, his father was, and now this new boy is not. It was never an issue—their different appearance— between my husband and his father, and I'd guess it won't be one for our son."

Today, the American Academy of Pediatrics maintains that there are no compelling medical reasons to circumcise baby boys.[20] The United States is the only country in the world that routinely performs this surgery for secular reasons. Like the risks associated with any surgery, possible risks of this procedure include pain, infection, bleeding, mutilation, interference with breastfeeding, and even death. The procedure includes strapping the baby into a special constraint, and too often it's done without any anesthesia. Don't be fooled into believing your baby won't feel any pain.

If you decide to leave your baby intact, know that he won't be alone. In the U.S. today, less than 60 percent of newborn boys are circumcised, and this rate has declined steadily over the last few decades. In other countries around the world, intact boys greatly outnumber circumcised boys.

If you decide to have your baby circumcised, the AAP recommends that anesthesia be used—and something more than just a topical cream.[21] You may want to follow the guidelines based on Jewish tradition, even if you aren't of Jewish faith. The procedure is performed on the eighth day after birth, when vitamin K levels are at their peak and the blood's clotting ability has kicked in. Your baby is never out of your presence, and you can comfort him throughout the procedure.

YOUR NEWBORN'S APPEARANCE, ABILITIES, AND BEHAVIOR

Your baby will take her time to stretch out of the fetal position—a pose she was in for so long. There's much for you to see as your baby unfolds her fingers, arms, and numerous creases in her skin. Her beautiful tiny fingernails and toenails may bring you hours of contemplation.

The biggest part of your newborn's body is her head. Labor and birth may have temporarily changed its shape (molding), but it'll regain a normal shape within days. She may have a blister on her head (caput) that developed when her head pressed against your cervix during labor. It'll eventually disappear.

She has tiny ears; silky, slicked down hair (if she has hair); and if the lighting isn't too bright, wide-open eyes that seek you out. The puffiness in her face will decrease now that she's out of the watery womb. Increased hormone levels at birth have made her genitals swollen, but the swelling will decrease as the hormones level off.

Your newborn will probably keep her hands closed into little fists, even while asleep. Her grasping reflex is so strong, you can help her pull herself into a sitting position. Even her little feet—with toes lined up like peas in a pod—try to grasp like hands when touched.

The following sections describe your baby's appearance, abilities, and behavior in more detail.

Skin and Sense of Touch

While your baby was in the womb, your body made vernix
(a creamy, white, lanolin-like substance) to cover and protect
her skin. She'll be born covered in a little or a lot of vernix.
(Some babies are born covered with more of it than others.)
Your baby's body may also still have lanugo, the downy hair
that covered her body while in the womb. It'll disappear
within a couple of days.

Your baby spent the last forty weeks comfortably and
safely immersed in amniotic fluid and covered in vernix.
After birth, there's no reason to wash away the vernix or the
scent of amniotic fluid. In fact, it's particularly important
that the fluid's scent stay on your baby's hands so she can
taste and smell it and connect the scent to the taste and scent
of your skin. Once born, she can be patted dry with warm
towels as she lies on your bare chest or abdomen. A lifetime
of baths and showers, soaps and towels, awaits her, but the
first precious moments should be spent touching and
connecting with you.

In the first couple of days after birth, your baby's skin
and the whites of her eyes may take on a yellowish tinge.
This coloring, called jaundice, is related to bilirubin levels
in her blood. Bilirubin is a pigment produced by the normal
breakdown of red blood cells in the liver, and it's discarded
in stool (poop). The normal process of eating and excreting
prevents bilirubin levels from becoming dangerously high.

Jaundice is common in babies because their livers are still
developing and removing extra red blood cells needed for
fetal circulation. The yellowish color will fade away naturally
within a week or two as your baby eats more and her liver
matures. A breastfed baby sometimes stay yellow a bit longer,
but this condition is absolutely normal. If your breastfed baby
is nursing well and gaining weight, there's no cause for concern.

To treat jaundice, some hospitals routinely place newborns
under a special ultraviolet light to help break down the
bilirubin in the skin. However, this procedure is rarely
necessary. In fact, some experts now believe that jaundice
may be a normal phenomenon in newborns.[22] To prevent
jaundice from becoming a problem, breastfeed your baby at

least ten to twelve times a day. The extra feedings of breast milk will help your baby excrete extra bilirubin in stool. You might also expose your baby to sunlight. Its ultraviolet rays work the same way as the hospital's artificial "bili-lights."

The skin is the body's largest sense organ, and babies thrive and develop best when their skin is touched. Not only does immediate and constant touching stimulate the production of growth hormones and aid the immune system, but it also helps establish better sleep patterns and prevent distress.

In the weeks ahead, carry your baby against you or in a sling or front carrier as often as you can. The contact will let you both learn how to respond to each other's signals and needs. Consider giving your baby a daily massage to relax and quiet yourselves together.

Mouth, Voice, and Sense of Taste

Your baby's mouth may look like a beautiful little rosebud. She'll use it to yawn, sneeze, cough, hiccup, and coo—all responses to her new environment and little rehearsals for life ahead. But from this perfect tiny orifice, she'll emit a mighty cry. A newborn's cry is nature's call, a universal summons for attention, and it's vital to her survival. At birth, some babies cry more than others, and some babies will require more attention in response to their cries than others. You may have seen a mother insert her pinky finger into her baby's mouth to quickly settle down the little one. This action helped meet two important needs: the need to be held and the need to suck.

The sucking and rooting reflexes are your baby's most important survival tools. Immediately after birth, she may begin to nudge (the rooting reflex) toward your nipples, which throughout pregnancy have darkened into "targets" she can see more easily. Your baby sucks in response to stress or fear, as well as for comfort and nutrition. During the first hours, sucking your breasts brings colostrum (the rich, clear "first milk" that's loaded with antibodies) into her little body. Her continued sucking eventually brings in your milk and helps your uterus contract more efficiently in the hours and days after the birth. Some babies are born ready to breastfeed right away. Some may need a little more time, choosing to nurse a little more sedately. If your baby's a strong nurser, it's common for a little blister to form on the inside of her upper lip.

Your baby was born able to taste. In fact, her taste buds were already developing when she was just eight weeks or so into gestation.[23] While in the womb, she tasted the spices, flavorings, and chemicals that you ate and absorbed then passed on to her through the placenta. During the first few months, she'll respond positively to only sweet flavors—and your breast milk is indeed sweet to the taste.

Eyes and Sense of Sight

© Marilyn Nolt

At birth, a newborn's eyes often appear red and puffy, and there may be broken blood vessels in the eyeballs, caused by pressure exerted on them during birth or by the drops or ointment she may have received after birth. Light-skinned babies usually have blue-gray eyes, and dark-skinned babies usually have brown eyes. Permanent color won't develop for about six months. Some babies can produce tears from birth, but most don't for six weeks or so.

The dark, beautiful orbs peering out from your newborn's face can see objects at close range (within eight to ten inches). Research shows that babies can recognize their mothers' faces in as little as four hours after birth. Your baby can even respond to your facial expressions, especially when you're within eight to ten inches of his face. Studies confirm that movement attracts babies' sight and newborns prefer curved shapes over straight ones, patterns in contrasting colors over plain patterns, and ordered patterns over random patterns. And they find the human face the most attractive thing to look at.[24]

Your baby's alertness at birth allows for her first "reading lesson"—assuming that no drugs were given during the birth process to dull his responses. As you and your baby gaze at each other, you're reading each other's cues, sending each other messages, making contact. Your baby may stare at you intently for long periods as he sorts through the surrounding stimuli. Or he may close his eyes, desiring a little more time before entering the bright, stimulating new environment. These hours of alert gazing send parents this important message: Pay attention!

Ears and Sense of Hearing

Months before your baby's birth, she can hear your internal body sounds as well as the sounds of the outside world—voices (especially yours), rumbling vehicles, ringing bells, barking dogs, sounds that surround us every day. Within the first hours of life, her tiny ears channel a great deal of information, helping her analyze and categorize the new surroundings.

Studies show that newborns prefer a live human voice over a recorded or telecast voice and an animated voice over an emotionally flat one.[25] Babies also prefer to be looked at while spoken to. When you instinctively speak directly to your newborn in a gentle, high-pitched voice, she listens and responds in recognition. She turns her head to the sound source, opens and brightens her eyes, and moves her arms and legs.

Nose and Sense of Smell

At birth, your newborn's nose appears flat and broad. Her brain's olfactory (smell) center formed very early in fetal development, so she likely has a sense of smell at birth. Her sense of smell (and taste) helps her reach your breast and nurse. Studies show that within a few days of birth, your baby can distinguish among the scent of your milk and other skin odors.[26] Certainly, your scents are the most familiar and comforting to your newborn—yet another important reason to not wash away amniotic fluid or vernix from her skin right after birth. It's also a good idea to wrap your baby in soft clothing that you've worn so your scent will comfort her.

Behavior

At birth, reactions to the new environment vary from baby to baby. If your baby isn't separated from you, he'll likely pensively and inquisitively stare at his new surroundings for an hour or much longer. If he's separated from you, he'll probably become distressed as he seeks the comfort of your skin to reassure him that he can trust these new surroundings.

Your newborn may begin vocalizing right away, making little grunts or whimpering rhythmically while staring at his new world. It's as though he's waiting to hear some familiar, gentle, and reassuring words and sounds he can respond to. Or your baby may be more reserved, seeking the safety and comfort of your arms a bit longer before more actively engaging with his surroundings. He may prefer silence or hushed voices and may be startled by noise, brightness, chatter, and bustle.

> Sarah remembers well the strong feeling of recognition that swept over her when her newborn son was placed in her arms: "He made these lovely little noises, and I had such an overwhelming desire to keep whispering to him, 'I know you! I know you!' It was as if we'd been together forever—like these wise little eyes staring into mine were familiar, and he recognized his father and me. I sort of assumed he expected to hear us welcoming him home."

Researchers have observed several states in newborn behavior. (See the following list.) Your baby's behavior will follow a pattern that'll develop at its own pace.[27]

- **Quiet alert state**: If any drugs given during the labor and birth haven't dulled her responses, your baby's first hour is one of attentiveness and quiet inquisitiveness. She focuses all her energy to look directly into your eyes and to listen to the surrounding voices. After this initial quiet alert state in the first hour of life, there are often few such prolonged periods over the next few days. Usually, briefer periods of curious, exploratory behavior occur around feeding time. In the first week of life, the normal baby spends only 10 percent of any twenty-four-hour period in this state.

- **Active alert state**: During this state baby is very different. He moves his arms and legs every two or three minutes (not continuously but rhythmically), makes small sounds, and looks around. These bursts of movements happen before feeding or when baby is fussy.

- **Crying state**: Crying is your baby's mode of communication. Her cry signals a need that you can learn to discern from other cries, such as recognizing "I'm hungry" from

"I need a diaper change." Pediatrician Marshall Klaus and his wife, Phyllis, have lovingly studied newborn behavior and encourage parents to recognize their newborn's different cries: "Sometimes it takes many tries to figure it out…. Holding the baby close, murmuring soothing words, and especially keeping oneself calm can be helpful in reading the baby's signals." Picking up your baby will often stop her crying, and research suggests that babies whose cries get responses quickly are less likely to cry at one year of age.[28]

- **Drowsy state**: This state occurs right before your baby drifts to sleep or right after she wakes up. It's similar to how you feel right before you fall into a nap on the couch, or just as you crawl out of bed in the morning in search of that first cup of coffee. In this state, your baby may continue to move a little as well as smile and frown.
- **Quiet sleep state**: A baby often drifts into this state at his mother's breast. It's deep and peaceful, with regular breathing, closed eyes, and few body movements.
- **Active sleep state**: In this state, your baby moves her eyes under closed eyelids, moves her arms and legs, speeds up her breathing, and displays a variety of endearing funny faces—goofy smiles, grimaces, and frowns—sometimes in quick succession. She tends to move or root around, as though seeking to get close to an edge or object. Babies will move toward the warmth, sound, and smell of their mothers' bodies in bed before they'll settle into quiet sleep.[29] When she wakes up, she's usually coming out of active sleep.

MORE ON BREASTFEEDING

It's in your baby's nature to find your breast and latch on to it himself. When he's hungry, he'll give you cues, the same ones he makes when he moves into the active sleep state. For example, he may appear asleep, but his eyes are moving beneath his lids and he moves his arms and hands to his mouth. He bobs his head from side to side and may even try to suck on your arm or face if you're holding him. He may make small noises. These actions are his natural way of alerting you that he's ready to find the breast, latch on, and suck. If you wait until he cries—which may be as long as thirty minutes after he starts giving you cues—he's no longer in a state to nurse easily. You'll have to settle him down before he's ready to feed.

In the first hours after birth it's easiest to let your baby position and latch on your breast himself. Hold him skin-to-skin vertically between your breasts, and let him bob his head and move until he finds your breast. Your baby will know your breast by feel and your nipple by smell, not by sight.

Or you can position your baby wrapped around you. Make sure he can move freely. Remove constricting blankets and uncover his hands. Snuggle your baby close, resting his head on your wrist or forearm, positioning him on his side facing you. He should be able to see your face with his top eye. His ear, shoulder, and hips should be in a straight line, and his nose should be level with your nipple. If you use a pillow, make sure you (not the pillow) are supporting your baby's body. As your baby nurses, support his neck and shoulders with your hand, but don't hold the back of his head.

Supporting him this way gives him the freedom to move his head. When he feels your breast against his chin and lower lip and smells your nipple, he'll open his mouth wide and move his upper lip up and over the nipple. This is an off-center (or asymmetric) latch, and it's the equivalent of you opening your mouth wide and placing the bottom of a very large hamburger on your lower lip, then moving your mouth up and over the top of the burger to stuff as much as possible into your mouth. If you approached the burger straight on, you couldn't fit nearly as much into your mouth, even if it's opened wide. The same logic holds true for your baby and the breast.

When eating that huge hamburger you also squeeze it to make it easier to bite. You can make your breast easier for your baby to latch onto by making a "breast sandwich." It helps to hold your breast with your index finger under your breast and your thumb on top. Then rotate your fingers so your breast rests in a U between your thumb and fingers. Your fingers and thumb are at three o'clock and nine o'clock. Now squeeze your breast to make a sandwich as your baby opens his mouth wide and latches on.

If your baby latches on properly, you shouldn't feel pain as he nurses, although most women experience some discomfort initially when their babies start sucking—just until their milk lets down. Whether your breasts feel full or not, your ducts release the milk only when your baby's sucking releases the hormone oxytocin. You'll know your milk has let down if your baby begins to suck differently (*suck, suck, suck* changes to *suck, swallow, suck, swallow*). You may relax, feel warm, or get thirsty. Or you may simply notice that your baby has settled down and is more content. In the first days after birth, you'll notice your uterus contracting as you nurse. Oxytocin is doing double duty: allowing your milk to "let down" and keeping your uterus tight.

Your baby will nurse happily until he's full, at which time he'll spontaneously release the breast. He may be sleeping, or he may want to continue nursing from the other breast. (If he isn't interested in the second breast, that's okay.) The hind milk, the milk at the end of a feeding, is very high in fat. It's important that your baby get the hind milk so he'll get the calories he needs and gain weight faster. The only way you can be sure your baby's getting the hind milk is if he finishes a feeding himself. Don't limit his time on the breast or insist that he take both breasts.

How often should you feed your baby? Feed him whenever he gives any cues that he's hungry and at least eight to twelve times a day. The more your baby nurses, the more milk you make. Don't delay a nursing session, and don't limit how long he nurses.

How will you know your baby's getting milk at each feeding? You'll know by noticing the change in his sucking.

He'll follow bursts of sucking with a pause as he swallows. You can also see his neck muscles move as he swallows.

At first, your baby gets colostrum from your breasts. His stomach is very small (the size of a walnut), and he doesn't need much of this very rich, clear liquid. Colostrum acts as a laxative, and your baby's first stool is the dark, tar-like meconium leaving his digestive system. Over the next two to four days, the color of his stool changes to a mustard yellow. The changing color of his stools is an important sign that he is getting your milk. Breastfed babies' stools are very watery, in part because there's so little waste—your baby's body can use almost everything in breast milk. Around the third day (sometimes sooner), your milk "comes in," and a feeling of fullness always accompanies it. Most women welcome this feeling as confirmation that they're actually making milk!

Ultimately, you'll know your baby's getting enough nutrition if he's gaining weight and wetting four to six disposable (or six to eight cloth) diapers and soiling at least three diapers in twenty-four hours. But it takes a few days for your baby to have this output. On day two he'll have two to three wet diapers and two stools, and over the next three days he'll work up to six wet diapers and at least three dirty diapers in a twenty-four–hour period.

Breastfeeding Help

We recommend several breastfeeding books and resources in Recommended Resources. For breastfeeding success, it's important that you have someone knowledgeable and experienced in the first weeks of nursing waiting in the wings in case you need help. The following are problems that are easily prevented and can be solved with simple solutions.

Engorgement

Engorgement is a painful condition in which the breasts become overly full with milk. Mothers whose babies are kept near so they can nurse frequently and efficiently in the first days don't become engorged. However, your breasts may become very engorged if your baby has had trouble latching and emptying your breasts in the first days, or if you've been separated from your baby. To prevent engorgement, keep your baby close and nurse frequently round the clock. To treat engorgement, have your baby nurse frequently. You may need to pump or hand-express some milk so your baby can latch on more easily. Or take a warm shower before nursing to help your milk begin dripping from your breasts and make your nipples softer. Once your baby's nursing, gently massage your breasts to encourage milk flow. Between feedings, ice may reduce swelling and pain. For more help, contact a lactation consultant.

Sore and Cracked Nipples

Your nipples shouldn't hurt when you nurse. If they do, it's almost always because your baby isn't latching on or sucking properly. It is important that you get help immediately. Don't wait. Contact a lactation consultant or someone knowledgeable about proper positioning and latch and have her watch you with your baby at the breast. She will help you with latch and position problems. As your nipples heal, once latch has been corrected, try changing your baby's position while nursing to move the pressure to an unaffected area. To help prevent cracked nipples, don't use soap to wash them—just use water and let them air-dry. Lanolin creams may help soothe sore nipples. Hydrogel pads (available from pharmacies) may also help relieve pain.

Baby Trouble

If your baby's sleepy because of medication you had in labor or is exhausted from the birth, he may not be interested in nursing during the first day or so, or he may have a lot of difficulty latching on and sucking. A lactation consultant can definitely help you. It's critical that your baby eat, and it's critical that milk is emptied from your breasts so you'll keep making more. If your baby hasn't had a successful nursing session in the first twelve hours, pump some colostrum and feed it to him with an eyedropper or small medicine cup. In most cases, there's no need to give him infant formula. Keep your baby skin-to-skin, pay attention to his feeding cues, and be patient—with yourself and with your baby.

BEYOND BABYMOON

The rush of your baby's birth is over, and now it's time to settle into being a family. At one time, women spent the days and weeks after giving birth lying in—an old term for that period of seclusion when a new mother concentrates on her newborn and is cared for by other women. Many traditional cultures have nurturing women who help care for the new mother and baby and manage the household. In traditional Jewish culture, for example, women care for a new mother entirely for the first thirty days after giving birth.

In our modern culture, in which so many women work outside the home and generations often don't live near one another, arranging a time for lying in can be difficult. Today's women expect (and are expected) to be independent and resilient, to jump back into prebirth routines in a slim, prebirth body, with every hair in place and appointments kept. This expectation makes women give the warped message *I'm back to normal! I'm good at this! Nothing has changed!* But becoming a mother does change a woman. Often a new mother doesn't realize that she needs nurturing just as much as her newborn does. She needs unrushed time and space to adjust to the transformation in her life.

To help make your time of adjustment easier, make some preparations before your baby's birth. Arrange for maternity leave, stock the freezer with premade meals, figure out what tasks you'll need help to do. These preparations can calm you and help you happily anticipate your baby's arrival. Once your baby's born, it's a time to relax obligations and rest. It's also a private, intimate, and emotional time that calls for protection and boundaries.

In a world where many feel isolated from one another, welcoming a new baby is a celebration friends and family long to attend. They're ready to admire the newborn, and encourage and congratulate the new parents. They're honored to arrange naming ceremonies, prepare special foods, take photographs, and give loads of gifts. Accept these gestures and encourage brief visits from well-wishers, but stay home and let them visit you—right in your bedroom, if necessary, where they can drink a cup of tea and admire you and your baby. Don't be shy asking visitors for help with dishes or laundry or any other task. Most will be eager to help. And don't worry about turning visitors away. Hang a "do not disturb" sign on your front door when you need to sleep and enjoy some privacy. Turn off your cell phones and land-line phones. Do whatever it takes to protect your quiet time with your new child.

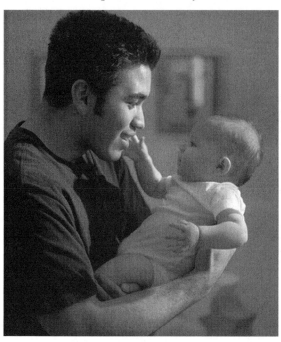

During the first hours and days with your newborn, let yourself surrender to unhurried, undivided time so you can get to know this new person who has changed—and will continue to change—your life profoundly. Sharpen your listening and observation skills to learn how best to respond to your little one. The cues and clues are there—you just need to act on them confidently, like the good parent you are.

Brian's transition to fatherhood was like Alice's trip through the looking glass: "There was an exact moment when Jonathan came into my arms, and all of a sudden I was a father. You can talk about it all of those months beforehand, but the reality doesn't really hit until the moment you're holding him." He and his wife, Susan, had their quiet, regimented apartment life thrown into temporary chaos, with family and friends dropping in with food and gifts, people gathered in the bedroom hour after hour, the constant kitchen clean-up taken up by this visitor or that. "At the end of the partying, there we were, the three of us, and Susan and I were exhausted on just about every level. And we found ourselves speaking to each other not only as husband and wife, like we had been just days before, but also as mother and father. It was—I don't know—a weird transition."

Chapter 13

_____

EARLY PARENTING

_____

Your children need your presence
more than your presents.
—Jesse Jackson

LIFE WITH YOUR NEWBORN

When your new baby arrives, you spend more time listening and learning than you ever had before. You focus all your attention on your little one, who has so much to teach you about caring for him. You learn more about parenting from each other than you ever could from any book or website. While with your baby, try to provide as quiet a setting as possible. It's difficult to learn his subtle behaviors in a setting with distractions.

Speaking of distractions, you may notice that you're receiving advice as never before—advice from family, friends, professionals, even strangers. Most advice is well meaning. But much of it is uninvited, some of it may hurt your feelings, and some of it is just plain misinformation.

Your relationship with your baby is unique, and together you're charting unknown waters. So when a friend tells you her secret for getting a baby to stop crying, or when Grandma suggests that

Getting advice often isn't easy, especially when the advice is about your ability to parent your child. When someone—particularly someone with whom you have an intense relationship, such as your mother or mother-in-law—gives you unsolicited advice on how to care for your baby, you may feel defensive, hurt, angry, judged, or inferior. The elevated levels of hormones in your postpartum body may keep you on edge for a while. A comment that you may have shrugged off before you got pregnant now stings.

To help you deal with unwelcome advice, repeat these affirmations to yourself:

- I have every reason to trust my own inner wisdom to care for this baby.
- I know my baby, and my ears are tuned in a special way to my child.
- I am wise enough to learn the dance that's begun between this unique child and me.

At the same time, simply thank the person offering the advice and change the subject or, if the person is determined to expound on the advice, excuse yourself and leave the room.

you put your baby on sleeping and eating schedules, you may need to turn a deaf ear. What worked for Baby Susie or was the norm forty years ago may not apply to you and your baby.

This chapter describes a way to parent your new child so he feels safe and secure. It discusses sleeping and feeding: two activities central to your baby's well-being. It also discusses your emotional and physical health after giving birth and becoming a mother, as well as changes to your lifestyle and household now that your baby has arrived.

ATTACHMENT PARENTING

Attachment parenting is a style of care that helps develop a child's trust, empathy, and affection. Its goal is to build a secure, enduring relationship between parent and child.

You probably practiced attachment parenting long before your baby was in your arms. When you caressed and spoke to your belly, you fostered loving attachments to your unborn baby. When you insisted that she stay with you once born, you continued to foster loving attachments to your newborn. And when your baby is at home, you have the opportunity to lovingly respond to her cues and signals, to her cries, and to things in her environment that might distress her. Just as your newborn thrives on touch in those first hours, your baby will continue to flourish when you stay close and respond to her. This style of parenting will continue to decrease stress levels for you and your baby, helping him relax and sleep and grow and learn.

There's a lot to learn when your baby comes home, but attachment parenting helps you learn these lessons naturally by keeping him close. The following two sections discuss how attachment parenting can help your baby get the sleep and nutrition she needs.

Sleep

Nighttime Feedings

Just as your baby's development in the womb guides you through pregnancy and birth, his verbal and physical cues and responses guide you through early parenthood. During the early weeks, your baby nurses frequently to nourish his rapidly growing body and keep up your milk supply. These round-the-clock feedings help you and your baby communicate better, and they regulate sleeping and waking patterns for you both.

Nighttime feedings are extra important. At night, breast milk is richer in important fats that the baby needs. And round-the-clock feedings maintain prolactin levels. High prolactin levels ensure excellent milk supply and decrease fertility. Many women relish the richness of these quiet nighttime feedings, when nothing distracts mother or baby from this special bonding.

Suzanne recalls those early weeks with her baby: "If I'd known how quickly those weeks would pass and how soon those times alone with my baby's dear little face looking up to me in the dimness of the night would end, I would have treasured the privilege even more. I would have whined less, I think, when I let tiredness bother me."

Sleep Schedules

Most parents of newborns and young babies long for a solid, uninterrupted night of sleep. Their own parents may advise, "Get that baby on a schedule so you can get some sleep!" But this advice is outdated and based on research done on formula-fed babies who had schedules imposed on them. Today, things are changing for the better. More and more babies are breastfed, and many share the same bed as their parents.

The research of James McKenna, PhD, director of the Mother-Baby Behavioral Sleep Laboratory at the University of Notre Dame, sheds light on the natural, typical sleep behaviors of babies and exposes the faulty research behind sleep schedules. Outside of North America, McKenna points out, parents don't consider their baby's unique sleep patterns as unusual or bothersome—they're normal for that baby. But in North America, parents are determined to get their babies to sleep, especially at night. Many see the baby's wakefulness as a problem, rather than a natural process. Some may even judge their parenting abilities by how well the baby sleeps in the early weeks and months.

McKenna concludes there's no universal answer when it comes to babies and sleep. A solution that works for one family may not work for another. Some babies are more easygoing and less demanding than others, and every family is different, with unique practices, challenges, and needs. Parents of sensitive babies or babies who are light sleepers might assume they're to blame if the babies don't sleep soundly. Any "expert" advice or programs often make these tired parents lose confidence, become frustrated, and mistrust their intuition and common sense.[1]

If you receive advice, criticism, or disapproval when your baby doesn't sleep at night, you may be tempted to try any "solution." Remember that your baby's wakefulness isn't a problem to fix. Instead, view the times he's awake as opportunities to get to know each other. By patiently accepting these early weeks and months of interrupted sleep—and understanding they're temporary—you reduce the pressure to get sleep at scheduled times. Babies usually sense when their parents (and environments) are more relaxed, so they relax more, too.

Cosleeping

Before the late 1700s, babies and mothers around the world slept together in the same bed. Around this time, in cultures affected by the Industrial Revolution (especially in Europe and North America), baby beds were introduced to families and soon become the norm. Today, the concept of cosleeping in a family bed is controversial. Some parents strongly feel their baby is safer and healthier when sleeping in a family bed. Others believe a family bed is unnatural, unsafe, and unhealthy.

Over the last two centuries, many cultures have forgotten the benefits of cosleeping—particularly North American culture, which has long stressed independent behavior in babies at earlier ages than in other cultures. But the popularity of cosleeping is growing, as medical and anthropological research shows that cosleeping promotes bonding and breastfeeding and perhaps prevents sudden infant death syndrome (SIDS).[2]

Just as skin-to-skin contact after birth benefits both newborn and mother, such close contact during the night also helps form stronger attachments between the two. Mother and baby sleep better because cries are met faster, which tends to

If you choose to sleep with your baby in a family bed, follow these safety guidelines:[3]

- Sleep on a flat, firm, and smooth mattress that's large enough to accommodate everyone comfortably. Don't sleep on a pillow-top mattress, waterbed, beanbag chair, or sofa.
- Make sure there isn't any space between the mattress and the bed frame or wall.
- Remove all pillows and heavy blankets during the early months. Use only a thin blanket for cover. Be very careful when adding pillows or blankets as your baby gets older.
- Make sure fitted sheets can't be pulled loose.
- As you dress your baby for sleep, keep in mind that body heat will add warmth during the night. Make sure your baby doesn't become overheated.
- Don't wear nightclothes with strings or long ribbons. Don't wear jewelry. If you have long hair, tie it up.
- Don't allow pets to sleep in the family bed with your baby.
- Put your baby on her back to sleep.
- Allow only one baby at a time in a family bed.
- Be wary of putting your baby in a family bed if you or anyone else is physically large. If there's a large dip in the mattress or if gravity makes your baby roll toward you while lying on the bed together, consider another sleeping arrangement.
- Do *not* put a baby in the family bed if you or anyone has used drugs or alcohol, is seriously sleep-deprived, or is smoking in the bed.
- Never leave your baby alone in an adult bed.

make a baby cry less. Research shows that when mother and baby rest together, their sleep is less disturbed.[4]

La Leche League International, a well-known breast-feeding organization, recommends cosleeping as a healthy way to feed and care for babies. James McKenna believes that babies who sleep with their mothers enjoy greater natural immunization from breastfeeding because they're free to nurse more frequently. Plus, cosleeping increases the number of night feeds, keeping prolactin levels high and delaying the onset of ovulation. The decreased fertility of breastfeeding women is dependent on keeping prolactin levels high around the clock.

When baby and mother sleep in the same bed, their body rhythms—including breathing patterns—synchronize. Some research shows that the shared sleep patterns and body rhythms may lower the risk of sudden infant death syndrome (SIDS).[5] A mother who's physically closer to her sleeping baby may sense when he's in trouble more quickly than if he were sleeping away from her.

Many cosleeping advocates believe that parents who sleep with their babies in the same bed are more confident and relaxed, eventually leading to more confident and relaxed children. Harvard University researcher Michael Commons found that babies who sleep alone might be more susceptible to stress disorders later on, with stress hormones actually causing physical changes in the brain.[6]

Despite the benefits of cosleeping, in 1999 the Consumer Product Safety Commission (CPSC) warned that putting a baby to sleep in an adult bed could be hazardous.[8]

When scientific studies confirm that babies benefit psychologically and physically from cosleeping, writer Jennifer Coburn wonders, "Why do parents flock to [stores] to purchase dolls that have heartbeats, sing lullabies, and snore when they can do the same for free?" She goes on to speculate that sleep disorders—rather than being part of a baby's biology—are actually created by well-intended parents who've bought into the idea of isolating a baby in a baby bed in the nursery, letting him cry himself to sleep so he learns to sleep independently. "Making one's self available by intercom is simply not meeting the nighttime needs of an infant," she writes. "It's time Americans join the rest of the world and parent our babies twenty-four hours a day."[7]

This warning, however, didn't explain that many deaths and accidents were the result of unsupervised babies who'd gotten trapped in the bed structure. The warning also failed to point out that some accidents and deaths were the result of an adult who'd used alcohol or drugs and rolled onto or smothered the baby. Furthermore, the warning was one-sided: it didn't mention the number of deaths or accidents that occurred in babies who slept alone and away from their parents.

Pediatrician and writer William Sears says, "On one hand, it is important to remind the parents who share a bed with their babies—and there are many—that they need to take certain precautions. On the other, these reports have unnecessarily frightened the millions of parents who safely and responsibly sleep with their babies." He concludes that when science and common sense don't match, perhaps faulty science and scientific reporting is to blame.[9]

Sleeping in the same bed may not be right for every family, but there are other ways to reap the benefits of cosleeping. Bedside co-sleepers or compact infant beds are perfect alternatives when sharing the same bed doesn't work. Some bedside co-sleepers can convert into freestanding bassinets, changing tables, and play yards.

CONTINUED BREASTFEEDING SUCCESS

Ideally, you and your baby are happily breastfeeding during the first days and weeks. However, it's not unusual for you to have some breastfeeding trouble—especially if you had a particularly rough labor and birth that led to the separation of you and your baby, who was fed formula or from a bottle.

For breastfeeding success, the instructions are simple: Keep your baby with you, respond to her feeding cues, position her so she comes "up and over" your nipple and areola, feed her at least eight to twelve times a day, and don't discourage her from feeding during the night. See pages 198–202 for more information.

Avoid giving your baby a bottle or a pacifier until breast-feeding is well established. Bottle nipples and pacifiers can cause problems with your baby's ability to suck at your breast. Plus, pacifiers can mask her early feeding cues, so she spends less time at the breast. Remember, the more time your baby spends at the breast in the first weeks, the more milk you produce.

While your body's making breast milk, remember you can eat and drink normally. There's no need to avoid spicy foods, foods that produce gas, or chocolate. Drinking caffeine and alcohol in moderation is usually just fine. You don't need to drink cow's milk to produce breast milk, and you don't need to drink gallons of water. Drink when you're thirsty and just enough to quench your thirst. It was once thought that breastfeeding women needed to drink large amounts of fluids to maintain milk supply. It was discovered, however, that women who drank fluids in excess when they weren't thirsty actually *decreased* milk production.[10]

Breast milk is the only food your baby should have for at least the first six months.[11] It's designed to provide all the nutrition she needs until she's ready to eat solid foods. Feeding her solids too soon only fills her with nutritionally inferior foods. Before they're six months old, most babies' digestive systems aren't developed enough to process solids effectively and safely, and many babies can't control their tongue and mouth muscles well enough to swallow solid foods safely.

Once your baby starts eating solid foods, breast milk should continue to be her main source of nutrition. The American Academy of Pediatrics recommends that babies consume breast milk for at least the first year,[12] and the World Health Organization extends this recommendation to the first two years.[13] The benefits of breastfeeding continue well beyond these recommended ages, and how long you continue to breastfeed your baby is a personal decision—one that's best made as your nursing relationship evolves. There's no need to decide early on how long you'll continue breastfeeding your child.

YOUR HEALTH

Symptoms of Emotional Distress

You've made it through forty weeks of pregnancy, with its nausea and weight gain. You've made it through the waiting and hard work of labor and birth. You now have a beautiful baby living with you—and you may be sad or depressed.

After giving birth, you'll experience emotional ups and downs. For some women, these emotional fluctuations are mild and subside within a few weeks. For others, they're overwhelming, long-lasting, and may require treatment. See page 214 to learn what's considered "normal" baby blues and what the symptoms are of postpartum mood disorders (PPMDs) and postpartum psychosis.

There's no clear scientific explanation for emotional distress after giving birth, although hormones, the environment, fatigue, and modern society have all been blamed. New mothers who've been treated for clinical depression before pregnancy may be more vulnerable to emotional distress. Some suggest the routine separation of newborns and mothers is a possible factor in the onset of emotional distress.

Just as having excellent support during labor can help a woman give birth confidently, having excellent postpartum support can help prevent a new mother from feeling overwhelmed and inadequate—emotions that can trigger sadness and depression if left unchecked. In many traditional cultures, family and friends care for and honor new mothers in the weeks and months after the babies' births. During this time, a new mother's only tasks are to nurse and get to know the baby. Before your baby's birth, try to find people you trust who can care for you during the days or weeks after your baby's birth. The support will better allow you to care for your baby—and better your chances of not slipping into a deep depression.

Baby Blues

Affecting 60 to 80 percent of new mothers, baby blues are temporary and rarely last longer than a week. Signs may include:

- Crying easily
- Feeling a loss of control
- Feeling a lack of confidence about being a parent
- Feeling overwhelmed
- Feeling exhausted, anxious, or sad

Postpartum Mood Disorders (PPMDs)

PPMDs occur within the first year after giving birth and can be long-lasting and require treatment. There are four different emotional conditions with their own signs:

Postpartum Anxiety and Panic Disorder

- Shortness of breath
- Lightheadedness
- Rapid heart rate
- Immobilizing fear of being alone, of dying, of baby dying
- Sensations of choking
- Faintness
- Chest pain
- Fear of leaving home

Postpartum Obsessive-Compulsive Disorder

- Repeated, uncontrollable thoughts, speech, and rituals that interfere with normal daily living

Postpartum Depression

- Affects about 10 to 20 percent of new mothers
- Loss of interest in everything
- Angry outbursts
- Sleeplessness
- Constant crying
- Fear of leaving home inadequacy, and low self-esteem
- Thoughts of harming self or baby
- Forgetting to eat or overeating

Postpartum Posttraumatic Stress Disorder

- Flashbacks
- Rage
- Anxiety
- Recurrent nightmares
- Extreme protectiveness
- Panic attacks

Postpartum Psychosis

Postpartum psychosis is rare but serious. Its signs may include:

- Severe agitation
- Depression
- Mood swings
- Delusion

If you're feeling sad or depressed as a new mother, rather than carrying these emotions by yourself amid raging hormones and demanding newborn care, ask your midwife, doula, or caregiver for help. He or she can suggest ways to help you move into a better state of mind and body. Here's what else you can do when you feel you're headed into sadness and depression:

- Share your feelings with others.
- Eat well and don't push yourself too hard. Find some peaceful moments, perhaps on a walk by yourself or in a warm bath.
- Try to sleep when your baby sleeps, or ask someone you trust to watch the baby so you can nap.
- Get some fresh air and sun, even if for just five or ten minutes.
- Relax your expectations. The laundry and dishes can wait. You can return phone calls and e-mails later. You need to concentrate on you and your baby now.
- Release your emotions rather than bottle them up. At times, being strong and staying controlled can do more psychological damage than letting go.

If your feelings of sadness and depression are not subsiding, or if you are experiencing any symptoms that point to more serious conditions, don't wait to get help. Get the help you deserve quickly.

Writer Anne Lamott writes about her journey into single motherhood in her memoir *Operating Instructions: A Journal of My Son's First Year.* In it, she chronicles the familiar emotional roller coaster she rode from day to day, and night to night, as a first-time parent groping her way through the challenges of caring for her infant son. "I'm crazy tired. I feel as stressed out by exhaustion as someone who spent time in Viet Nam." Every woman has her own, specific reasons for feeling as she does, especially in the weeks after birth. *Mothering* magazine editor Peggy O'Mara reminds us that depression needs to be acknowledged. "Don't allow anyone, including yourself, to downplay your emotional experience."

Your Body

Many women have described their postpartum bodies with honor, humor, or horror—for example, "Earth Mother," "Mama Bod," the "meltdown." You may have heard other terms, or even thought up some of your own after seeing a woman shortly after she's given birth.

The time it takes a new mother to settle into her true postpartum shape and weight varies greatly from woman to woman. To help keep your body healthy and energized and to help keep up milk production, continue to eat a healthy, balanced diet. Keep in mind that much of your pregnancy weight will slowly but surely disappear as you breastfeed over the next several months.

Seek balance and moderation as you resume your prepregnancy activities. Don't rush your body into its postpartum shape and weight. Remember, it took forty weeks for your body to change during pregnancy—it'll likely take at least that long to change completely once again. Before starting a high-exertion exercise program, wait until your postpartum bleeding has stopped. Meanwhile, walk as much as you can. This gentle, invigorating activity is one that you can do with your baby, that gets you out of the house, and that helps you get back in shape.

Author Kristin Beck found that she loved her body more after her baby's birth than before she became pregnant. "Yes, I'm bigger and stretchier and jigglier...but in the meantime I made a whole other person! I stand taller now and walk with greater purpose. I'm proud of my baby body, knowing that it gave my son a comfy vessel in which to gestate and [has been] the source of all his nourishment since birth."[14]

Contrary to the messages our culture conveys to us through different media, no one body type defines beauty. Beautiful women come in all shapes and sizes. In your postpartum journey, trust your body to find its true shape and size as mother of your baby.

Your Sex Life

When, where, and how a new mother resumes her sex life varies greatly from woman to woman. Some women are physically and emotionally ready to have sex within weeks after giving birth, and some need more time. Some women and their partners may be so tired or focused on parenting a newborn that lovemaking is the last thing on their minds. Others may have trouble meshing their sexual roles with their new roles as parents. Still others may have difficulty adapting to the woman's changed body.

Becoming lovers again after becoming parents can take time. Talk to each other, share your concerns and questions, be patient and understanding of each other, and don't hurry to resume the sexual activity you had before you became pregnant. Words and caresses can be empowering and healing—and sexy.

> Breastfeeding can decrease fertility. If you breastfeed exclusively and nurse at least once at night, you likely won't ovulate. Exclusive, round-the-clock breastfeeding is 98 percent effective in preventing pregnancy during the first six months. When your baby begins to eat solid foods, your fertility gradually returns—slowly, if you introduce solids slowly. Keep in mind, though, that breastfeeding doesn't guarantee you won't ovulate. If you're not ready for another pregnancy (and your body needs a rest between pregnancies), use common sense when having sex after your baby arrives.

To help your sex life adjust to your life as a new mother, remember to eat well, get rest, and look after your physical, emotional, and relationship needs.

OTHER CONCERNS AFTER THE BABY ARRIVES

Managing Your Household

Was your kitchen counter clutter-free before the baby arrived? Is there a layer of grime on top of your refrigerator? Is your laundry piling up? Does your partner apparently not see—or care about—the stack of junk that's been growing on the coffee table for so long?

If you're someone whose home was in perfect order before your baby's birth, it probably isn't after his arrival—and that's okay. Like many, many new mothers, your priorities have shifted. Vacuuming the rug and dusting the furniture become unnecessary. Instead, taking care of your baby's needs is first on your priority list. And this is the way it should be, as you welcome your little one into your family.

During the first few weeks, friends and relatives may give you advice or criticism on the state of your home. Their comments may make you question your ability to keep on top of things. If you can't keep a tidy home now, when your baby is small, how will you ever manage when he's older? Like unwanted advice, self-criticism can make you expend too much energy and wear yourself out over the wrong stuff, which makes you lose valuable learning and loving time with your baby.

Flash forward in your mind to a time when your newborn is now grown and moving out of your home to start adult life. Would you lament, "If only I'd kept my home cleaner and spent less time with him when he was a newborn"? Of course you wouldn't. This time with your new baby is fleeting, and it'll never be repeated. If you have to choose between getting the house in shape for Aunt Harriet's visit or rocking your baby as you listen to his sweet sounds, Aunt Harriet will just have to push aside the pile of towels to sit on your sofa. The time with your newborn is just too precious to waste, especially on housework.

However, at the very time when you least want to think about housework—and have little energy to do it—a disorganized household can overwhelm you. The best way to reduce stress in this area is to lower your expectations. Remember that you just can't do it all, and that caring for your baby, yourself, and the rest of your family is more important than having a spotless home. Another useful strategy: Analyze your household needs before your baby's birth and plan ahead to meet those needs. Putting a system in place can prevent arguments, keep your household running smoothly, and save you from managing all the details.

Deciding Whether to Return to Work

The decision of whether to return to work after having a baby is one of the most difficult choices many new mothers have to make. They base their decisions on financial, intellectual, or social reasons. Before your baby arrives, you may think you know your decision. But it's wise not to consider it set in stone—once your baby's born, you may have a change of heart. Writer and publisher Peggy O'Mara points out that a woman who's eight months pregnant can't imagine how she'll feel once the baby is born: "Some women simply never expect to be so in love with their babies."

Thanks to the Family and Medical Leave Act of 1993 (FMLA), many parents can stay home for at least a short time when they have a new child without losing ground at work. The FMLA requires certain employers to grant an eligible employee a twelve-week unpaid leave upon the birth or adoption of a child and to restore the employee to the same or an equivalent job at the end of the leave. For more information on the FMLA, contact the nearest office of the Wage and Hour Division, listed in most directories under *U.S. Government, Department of Labor*, or visit http://www.dol.gov/esa/whd/fmla.

When she became pregnant, Amy Bowan was young and just starting to climb the ranks as a technical writer for a software company. She planned to hire a nanny to care for her baby after a twelve-week maternity leave so she could return to work. "I brought home half the bacon in the family, and my career aspirations were just as important as my husband's," she said. She made all the necessary preparations for her absence at work.

After the birth, she began her nanny search, but "every time I looked at my baby, grief washed over me. The idea of leaving her, even for only twenty-four hours a week as I planned, sent me into a spiral of depression." A nanny was eventually hired, and Amy started back to work. She quickly learned that her husband would have to hand the baby over to the nanny in the mornings; she simply didn't have the heart to do it.

At work, Amy couldn't talk to others about her baby because it made her too sad. It took only a couple of weeks for her to make the choice to quit her job and care for her baby. "Didn't my baby deserve to wake up every morning knowing that someone who thought the world of her was going to spend the next twelve hours doing nothing but soak up every smile?" When she finds herself thinking about putting her career goals on hold, she's quick to respond, "I am grateful every day that I made the decision I did."

You may decide that when it comes to your baby's care, no one can replace you. Staying at home with your baby can be rewarding, fulfilling, exciting, and even fun, but it's definitely not easy (see page 221). The daily baby- and house-related chores and errands can be difficult to manage, as can the loss of income.

As you analyze your family's budget to see whether stay-at-home parenting is possible for you, include not only the cost of childcare, but also the cost of transportation to and from work, work clothing costs, and food costs while at work. These costs may make returning to work less cost-efficient than caring for your baby yourself. Organizations like Alternatives for Simple Living offer ways to live on less, and there are many books and websites on the subject as well. As writer Josh Hinds says, "Wealth comes in many forms, certainly not just monetary ones." Your baby is definitely a gift that's worth investing your time and effort.

With this said, however, it may just be impossible for you or your partner to care for your baby full-time. You may want to consider flexible employment options (see sidebar below for more information). If both of you must return to work, find and arrange suitable childcare well before your baby's birth. Formal daycare (daycare centers and home daycares) as well as informal daycare (nanny, au pair, babysitter, or a friend or relative) come with a host of challenges and concerns for you to consider, including certification documentation, safety procedures and record, and care styles, to name just a few.

Whatever childcare provider you decide to use, prepare your own interview questions, including ones that ask how the provider handles problems with sickness or behavior. Ask for references and follow up on them. Visit the sites a few times to observe how the provider and any staff members interact with children. Make at least one visit unannounced.

Each type of childcare has advantages and disadvantages. You must weigh the pros and

Some parents balance childcare and household management with income-producing work by staggering their schedules or working at home or part-time. Here are some flexible employment options you may want to investigate:

- Sharing a full-time job with another employee (job-sharing)
- Working at a job that's designed to be part-time
- Working weekends, nights, and/or evenings
- Working flexible hours (according to your employer's and family's needs)
- Working a compressed workweek
- Seasonal work
- Substitute or backup employment
- Working odd jobs
- Working someplace where your child can accompany you
- Working at home

cons of each before choosing the childcare that best ensures your baby's safety and well-being, meets your family's needs and budget, and gives you peace of mind.

Making Stay-at-Home Parenting Work

If you (or your partner) decide to stay at home with the baby, talk to other stay-at-home parents so you know what to expect. Analyze your financial situation to see whether your family's budget can support having a stay-at-home parent. If stay-at-home parenting is possible for you, make adult interactions part of your daily schedule. Network with other stay-at-home parents, or parents who work part-time. Keep in mind that it's essential for your baby's development—and your sanity—to get out of the house and let the world stimulate you both.

What does your heart tell you when you think about going back to the workplace right now? What does your heart tell you about your baby being cared for by someone other than you or your partner? What does your heart tell you about the things you value most in this part of your life? Answer these questions honestly, and your decision will never be wrong.

Pumping Breast Milk

If you're breastfeeeding your baby, at some point you may want to have someone else feed him—whether so you can enjoy an evening on the town with your partner or so you can return to work. This means that you'll need to be able to pump your breast milk and store it. It's a challenge to continue to breastfeed when you and your baby are apart, but many women do it and do it successfully.

The longer you can put off starting to pump your milk, the better your milk supply will establish itself. Try to allow yourself at least four months before starting to pump, to get to know your baby and develop confidence in your ability to parent him. When you return to work, try to arrange for a part-time schedule for the first few weeks, if possible.

Don't even think about pumping and storing your breast milk until about two weeks before returning to work. Until then, just enjoy your baby and work on making a good milk supply. This means nursing frequently around the clock. Two weeks before your return to work, start pumping after one daytime feeding and store the milk. As the week progresses, increase pumping to after two daytime feedings. The week before your return, leave your baby with someone you trust for a short time and have that person give your baby a bottle of your breast milk. A baby almost always drinks from a bottle more willingly if someone other than his mother gives him the bottle.

When you return to work, your employer should know that women employees who continue to breastfeed take less time off because their babies get sick less often. Investigate your company's policy and attitudes, as well as your legal rights, regarding breastfeeding. Make arrangements for expressing milk during the workday, including break time; privacy; a pump (manual or electric; borrowed, rented, or bought), collection kit, and storage supplies; and a safe storage place for milk. The more comfortable the setting is where you pump, the more easily your milk can let down. Express milk a couple of times during the day at preset times, taking extra care to keep the pump and bottles clean and the milk cold.

Breastfeeding organizations like La Leche League International (see Recommended Resources) provide wonderful information for nursing mothers to help with breastfeeding problems or questions—and for employers to learn the importance of pumping breast milk at work. Most breast-feeding books offer guidelines for working and breastfeeding. Talk to women who have successfully combined working and breastfeeding. Giving your baby breast milk while separated from him helps maintain all the benefits breast milk provides—even when you're not there to give it to him.

Handling Sibling Rivalry

If you have other children, know that no two children respond the same way to the arrival of a new brother or sister. Some may find the new baby exciting and want to help with baby care. Others want nothing to do with this strange interloper. Sibling rivalry is not surprising, especially when an older sibling is still very young. At this age, the child won't want to share your time and affection with another child.

When your baby first comes home, your older child may suddenly demand that you hold, carry, or feed her, especially when you're busy attending to the baby. Or your child may regress to baby behavior— sucking her thumb, wetting herself, speaking baby talk. She may even act aggressively, handling the baby roughly or striking at you.

Can you prevent sibling rivalry? Preparing your child before the baby's birth is a good start. Talk about your pregnancy to your child, involving her in the birth preparations as much as possible. Read together a children's book about being a big sister or brother. Arrange to spend some time around other babies. Share photos of your child's birth and infancy so she knows how you celebrated and treasured her own first year.

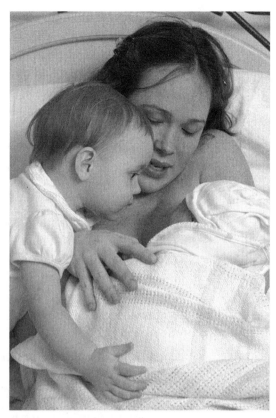

When the baby comes home, here are some suggestions for keeping your older child on an even keel:

- Introduce your child to the baby as soon as possible, preferably with no other visitors present.
- Spend (and see that your partner spends) some uninterrupted one-on-one time with your child every day.
- Change your child's routine as little as possible. Make any big changes (a new bed or bedroom, a new play group, a new babysitter) several months before or after the birth.
- Listen carefully to your child's feelings about the baby and the changes in your family. Help your child put his or her feelings into words if necessary. Acknowledge negative feelings—never deny or discount them.
- Make sure your child understands that absolutely no hurting is allowed. Give your child safe ways to express negative feelings, like drawing angry pictures, acting out with dolls, or roaring like a lion.

- Baby your child if she seems to need it. Don't worry about regression, which is likely to be short-lived. Expect less independence, and you're likely to get more.
- Make sure your child has some private space and things that she doesn't have to share with the baby.
- Give your child special jobs to help the family and the baby, but don't overdo it—take your cues from your child.
- Point out the benefits of being an older child, like choosing what to eat, being able to go the park and play, and having friends.

Despite all the preparations to avoid sibling rivalry, your older child will probably act out at least once if she feels her baby sibling is hogging the limelight. You may find it difficult at times to find the flexibility and calmness to handle her, but she needs a good long hug and some loving words from you to let her know you love her just as much as ever.

YOUR BABY, YOURSELF

In the weeks and months after giving birth, you'll find yourself dealing with many firsts with your baby. His first sickness, first teething, first baffling behavior you don't feel quite equipped to handle. You'll have to make decisions on issues that you've never thought about. You'll have to figure out how to integrate your prebaby life into your postbaby life—if that's even possible.

There'll be times when you won't find answers to a pressing question or concern about your baby—not in a book or a website, not from a friend or relative. There'll be sleepless nights and times when you feel as though you're not a good enough parent.

Parenthood can be one of life's greatest challenges and, at the same time, one of life's greatest blessings. It has the potential to make you a more complete person. Parenthood helps you learn to trust your instincts and believe in your strengths.

Fred Rogers—that wise, gentle parent and TV personality who modeled a deep trust and respect for children of all ages—once said: "Please think of the children first. If you

ever have anything to do with
their entertainment, their food,
their toys, their custody, their
day or night care, their health
care, their education—listen
to the children, learn about
them, learn from them. Think
of the children first."[15]

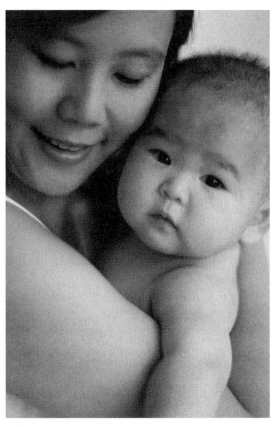

Remember that your baby
is always teaching you new
things about yourself. Your
role as a parent will grow and
change daily—sometimes
subtly; other times, dramatically. There'll be times when
you feel elated, as though
you're doing everything
right. And there'll be
times when your baby
has frustrated or exhausted
you beyond reason.

Be kind to yourself,
especially when your
parenting skills disappoint you, when you feel as if you
simply have nothing more to give, or when you find yourself
judging or shaming yourself. Remember that you and your
baby are learning the steps of a new dance together, and you
will make mistakes.

Parenting is an intense, intimate business, full of responsibilities and hard work. It's a crucial job that our world
depends on for the development of confident, conscientious
children who will one day follow in our footsteps. May the
journey ahead with your new child be one of gentle discovery,
patient giving, and boundless joy.

AFTERWORD

A baby is God's opinion that
the world should go on.
—Carl Sandburg

If you're pregnant as you read these words, you're a privileged woman. *Privilege* is defined as a special right or an opportunity to do something regarded as a special honor. No matter what your income, your education, your social status, your appearance, or your circumstances, you're privileged when you do the work of growing and birthing a baby.

For you, the hard work that lies ahead isn't just coping with labor pain or pushing a baby out. The hard work is resisting the inertia of "what is" in modern birth. When, for you and your baby's sake, you choose a normal, natural birth, you're choosing the road less traveled.

But it's not an untraveled road. Countless women have come to trust their bodies as they made choices about the *where, who, when,* and *what* of their births. Seek out their stories and find what you can learn from them. Midwife Ina May Gaskin says that birth stories like these share a world of wisdom, inspiration, and information: "Positive stories shared by women who have had wonderful childbirth experiences are an irreplaceable way to transmit knowledge of a woman's true capacities in pregnancy and birth."

Your own story will add to the history of strong, confident women who have approached birth as a normal, natural part of who they are. We hope the basic information we've shared in these pages has awakened your awareness of your own strength and wisdom—the strength and wisdom every woman carries.

You know what to do. You are beautifully and perfectly designed to give birth. You are not alone. May your choices, your story, your capabilities, and your strengths be an inspiration to other birthing women.

Appendix A
EFFECTIVE CARE IN PREGNANCY
AND CHILDBIRTH: A SYNOPSIS

Murray Enkin, MD, FRCS(C), LLD
Marc J.N.C. Keirse, MD, DPhil, DPH, FRANZCOG, FRCOG
James Neilson, BSc, MD, FRCOG
Caroline Crowther, MD, DCH, DDU, FRCOG, FRANZCOG
Lelia Duley, MD, MSc (Epid), MRCOG
Ellen Hodnett, RN, PhD
G. Justus Hofmeyr, MBBCH, MRCOG

EDITOR'S NOTE: *This article is the text and six tables from the final chapter (Chapter 50) of the new third edition of* A Guide to Effective Care in Pregnancy and Childbirth. *It summarizes the authors' conclusions and recommendations, based on the information they have compiled in the book about the beneficial or harmful effects of the various elements of care used during pregnancy and childbirth. The chapter numbers refer the reader to the relevant chapter of the book. (BIRTH 28:1 March 2001)*

The underlying thesis of this book is that evidence from well-controlled comparisons provides the best basis for choosing among alternative forms of care in pregnancy and childbirth. This evidence should encourage the adoption of useful measures and the abandonment of those that are useless or harmful.

In this final chapter we have tried to summarize the main conclusions reached in earlier chapters. This summary takes the form of six tables which list, respectively:

(1) beneficial forms of care;
(2) forms of care that are likely to be beneficial;
(3) forms of care with a trade-off between beneficial and adverse effects;
(4) forms of care of unknown effectiveness;
(5) forms of care that are unlikely to be beneficial;
(6) forms of care that are likely to be ineffective or harmful.

Tables 1 and 6 are based on clear evidence from systematic reviews of randomized controlled trials. Tables 2 and 5 are based on information from reviews of controlled trials or good observational evidence, but for which the conclusions cannot be as firmly based as those for Tables 1 and 6. Table 3 lists forms of care with both beneficial and adverse effects, which women and caregivers should weigh according to their individual circumstances and priorities; and Table 4 lists forms of care for which there are insufficient data, or data of inadequate quality on which to base a recommendation.

We have tried to be explicit about our criteria for choosing which table to use for each intervention, but there is inevitably some subjectivity in our choice. We worked from two basic principles: first, that the only justification for practices that restrict a woman's autonomy, her freedom of choice, and her access to her baby, would be clear evidence that these restrictive practices do more good than harm; and second, that any interference with the natural process of pregnancy and childbirth should also be shown to do more good than harm. We believe that the onus of proof rests on those who advocate any intervention that interferes with either of these principles.

A tabulated summary such as this is necessarily selective. Nuances discussed in the chapters cannot find full expression in summary tables. Nevertheless, we hope that the explicit form in which these conclusions have been stated will be useful, and that the advantages of this summary approach will outweigh its drawbacks.

The inclusion of a particular form of care in Tables 1 or 2 does not imply that it should always be adopted in practice. Research based on the study of groups may not always apply to individuals, although it should be relevant to guide broad policies of care. Forms of care listed in Tables 5 and 6 may still be useful in particular circumstances, although, once again, they should be discouraged as a matter of policy. Practices listed in Table 3 will require careful consideration by the individuals concerned, while those in Table 4 should usually be avoided except in the context of trials to better evaluate their effects.

Some of the conclusions that we have reached will be controversial, but they must be judged in the light of the methods we used to assemble and review the evidence on which they are based. While we have made great efforts to ensure that the data presented are comprehensive and accurate, it is possible that errors and misinterpretations have crept in. We conclude by reiterating the invitation extended to readers in our first edition, to bring omissions and mistakes to our attention for inclusion and correction in *The Cochrane Library* and in later editions of this book. Correspondence should be addressed to the Cochrane Pregnancy and Childbirth Group, Liverpool Women's Hospital NHS Trust, Crown Street, Liverpool, UK L8 7SS.

Table 1. Beneficial Forms of Care

Effectiveness demonstrated by clear evidence from controlled trials *Chapter*

Basic care

Women carrying their pregnancy record to enhance their feeling of being in control	3
Pre- and peri-conceptional folic acid supplementation to prevent recurrent neural tube defects	5, 6
Folic acid supplementation (or high folate diet) for all women envisaging pregnancy	5, 6
Assistance (especially behavioral strategies) to stop smoking during pregnancy	5
Balanced energy and protein supplementation when dietary supplementation is required	6
Vitamin D supplementation for women with inadequate exposure to sunlight	6
Iodine supplementation in populations with a high incidence of endemic cretinism	6

Screening and diagnosis

Doppler ultrasound in pregnancies at high risk of fetal compromise	12

Pregnancy problems

Antihistamines for nausea and vomiting of pregnancy that is resistant to simple measures	13
Local imidazoles for vaginal candida infection (thrush)	13
Local imidazoles instead of nystatin for vaginal candida infection (thrush)	13
Magnesium sulphate rather than other anticonvulsants for treatment of eclampsia	15
Administration of anti-D immunoglobulin to Rh-negative women whose newborn baby is not Rh-negative	18
Administration of anti-D immunoglobulin to Rh-negative women at 28 weeks of pregnancy	18
Antiretroviral treatment of HIV-infected pregnant women to prevent transmission to fetus	19
Antibiotic treatment of asymptomatic bacteriuria	19
Antibiotics during labor for women known to be colonized with group B streptococcus	19
Tight as opposed to too strict or loose control of blood sugar levels in pregnant diabetic women	20
External cephalic version at term to avoid breech birth	22
Corticosteroids to promote fetal maturity before preterm birth	25
Offering induction of labor after 41 completed weeks of gestation	26

Childbirth

Physical, emotional, and psychological support during labor and birth	28, 35, 41
Continuous support for women during labor and childbirth	28
Agents to reduce acidity of stomach contents before general anesthesia	29
Complementing fetal heart rate monitoring in labor with fetal acid-base assessment	30
Oxytocics to treat postpartum hemorrhage	33
Prophylactic oxytocics in the third stage of labor	33
Active versus expectant management of third stage of labor	33

Problems during childbirth

Absorbable instead of non-absorbable sutures for skin repair of perineal trauma	36
Polyglycolic acid sutures instead of chromic catgut for repair of perineal trauma	36

Techniques of induction and operative delivery

Prostaglandins to increase cervical readiness for induction of labor	39
Amniotomy plus oxytocin for induction of labor instead of either amniotomy alone or oxytocin alone	40
Vacuum extraction instead of forceps when operative vaginal delivery is required	41
Antibiotic prophylaxis (short course or intraperitoneal lavage) with cesarean section	43

Care after childbirth

Use of surfactant for very preterm infants to prevent respiratory distress syndrome	44
Support for socially disadvantaged mothers to improve parenting	45
Consistent support for breastfeeding mothers	46
Personal support from a knowledgeable individual for breastfeeding mothers	46
Unrestricted breastfeeding	46
Local anesthetic sprays for relief of perineal pain postpartum	47
Cabergoline instead of bromocriptine for relief of breast symptoms in non-breastfeeding mothers	48

Table 2. Forms of Care Likely to Be Beneficial

The evidence in favor of these forms of care is strong,
although not established by randomized trials   *Chapter*

Basic care
Adequate access to care for all childbearing women   3
Social support for childbearing women   3
Financial support for childbearing women in need   3
Legislation on paid leave and income maintenance during maternity or parental leave   3
Midwifery care for women with no serious risk factors   3
Continuity of care for childbearing women   3
Antenatal classes for women and their partners who want them   4
Advice to avoid excessive alcohol consumption during pregnancy   5
Avoidance of heavy physical work during pregnancy   5

Screening and diagnosis
Ultrasound to resolve questions about fetal size, structure, or position   8
Selective use of ultrasound to assess amniotic fluid volume   8
Selective use of ultrasound to estimate gestational age in first and early second trimester 8, 9
Ultrasound to determine whether the embryo is alive in threatened miscarriage   8, 14
Ultrasound to confirm suspected multiple pregnancy   8, 17
Ultrasound for placental location in suspected placenta previa   8, 21
Second trimester amniocentesis to identify chromosomal abnormalities in pregnancies at risk   9
Transabdominal instead of transcervical chorionic villus sampling   9
Genetic counseling before prenatal diagnosis   9
Clinical history to assess risk of pre-eclampsia   10
Regular monitoring of blood pressure during pregnancy   10
Testing for proteinuria during pregnancy   10
Uric acid levels for following the course of pre-eclampsia   10
Fundal height measurements during pregnancy   12

Pregnancy problems
Ultrasound to facilitate intrauterine interventions   8, 9
Antacids for heartburn of pregnancy if simple measures are ineffective   13
Bulking agents for constipation if simple measures are ineffective   13
Local metronidazole for symptomatic trichomonal vaginitis after the first trimester   13
Antibiotics for symptomatic bacterial vaginosis   13
Antiplatelet agents to prevent pre-eclampsia   15
Antihypertensive agents to control serious hypertension in pregnancy   15
Calcium to prevent pre-eclampsia, for women at high risk or with low calcium in diet   6, 15
Balanced protein/energy supplementation for impaired fetal growth   6, 16
Ultrasound surveillance of fetal growth in multiple pregnancies   17
Screening all pregnant women for blood group isoimmunization   18
Anti-D immunoglobulin to Rh-negative women after any uterine bleeding,
    intrauterine procedure, or abdominal trauma during pregnancy   18, 21
Intra-uterine transfusion for a severely affected iso-immunized fetus   18
Advice to not breastfeed for HIV-infected women to prevent transmission to baby   19, 46
Routine screening for, and treatment of, syphilis in pregnancy   19
Rubella vaccination of seronegative women postpartum   19
Screening for and treatment of chlamydia in high prevalence populations   19
Cesarean section for active herpes (with visible lesion) in labor with intact membranes   19
Prepregnancy counseling for women with diabetes   20
Specialist care for pregnant women with diabetes   20
Home instead of hospital glucose monitoring for pregnant women with diabetes   20
Ultrasound surveillance of fetal growth for pregnant women with diabetes   20
Allowing pregnancy to continue to term in otherwise uncomplicated diabetic pregnancies   20

Table 2. Continued

The evidence in favor of these forms of care is strong, although not established by randomized trials	*Chapter*
Careful attention to insulin requirements postpartum	20
Encouraging diabetic women to breastfeed	20
Checking for clotting disorders with severe placental abruption	21
Vaginal instead of cesarean delivery for placental abruption in the absence of fetal distress	21
Vaginal instead of cesarean birth for a dead fetus after placental abruption	21
Repeat ultrasound scanning of a low-lying placenta in late pregnancy	21
Delaying planned cesarean section for placenta previa until term	21
Cesarean section for placenta previa covering any portion of the cervical os	21
Ultrasound examination for vaginal bleeding of undetermined origin	21
External cephalic version for transverse or oblique lie at term	22
Tocolysis for external cephalic version of breech, particularly if unsuccessful otherwise	22
External cephalic version for breech in early labor if the membranes are intact	22
Corticosteroid administration after prelabor rupture of the membranes preterm	23
Vaginal culture after prelabor rupture of the membranes preterm	23
Antibiotics for prelabor rupture of the membranes with suspected intrauterine infection	23
Not stopping spontaneous labor after prelabor rupture of the membranes preterm	23
Elective delivery for prelabor rupture of the membranes preterm with signs of infection	23
Amnioinfusion for fetal distress thought to be due to oligohydramnios in labor	23, 30
Betamimetic tocolysis to allow effective preparation for preterm birth	24
Short-term indomethacin to stop preterm labor	24
Offering induction of labor as an option after fetal death	27
Prostaglandin or prostaglandin analogs for induction of labor after fetal death	27

Childbirth

Respecting women's choice of companions during labor and birth	28
Respecting women's choice of place of birth	28
Presence of a companion on admission to hospital	29
Giving women as much information as they desire	29
Freedom of movement and choice of position in labor	29
Change of mother's position for fetal distress in labor	30
Intravenous betamimetics for fetal distress in labor to "buy time"	30
Respecting women's choice of position for the second stage of labor and giving birth	32
Guarding the perineum versus watchful waiting during birth	32
Intramyometrial prostaglandins for severe postpartum hemorrhage	33

Problems during childbirth

Regular top-ups of epidural analgesia instead of top-ups on maternal demand	34
Maternal movement and position changes to relieve pain in labor	34
Counter-pressure to relieve pain in labor	34
Superficial heat or cold to relieve pain in labor	34
Touch and massage to relieve pain in labor	34
Attention focusing and distraction to relieve pain in labor	34
Music and audio-analgesia to relieve pain in labor	34
Epidural instead of narcotic analgesia for preterm labor and birth	34, 37
Amniotomy to augment slow or prolonged labor	35
Continuous subcuticular suture for perineal skin repair	36
Primary rather than delayed repair of episiotomy breakdown	36
Delivery of a very preterm baby in a center with adequate perinatal facilities	37, 44
Presence of a pediatrician at a very preterm birth	37, 44
Trial of labor after previous lower segment cesarean section	38
Trial of labor after more than one previous lower segment cesarean section	38

Table 2. Continued

The evidence in favor of these forms of care is strong, although not established by randomized trials	*Chapter*
Use of oxytocic agents when indicated for labor after a previous cesarean section	38
Use of epidural analgesia in labor when needed after previous cesarean section	38

Techniques of induction and operative delivery

Assessing the state of the cervix before induction of labor	39
Transverse instead of vertical skin incision for cesarean section	42
Low-dose heparin with cesarean section to prevent thrombo-embolism	42
Transverse lower segment uterine incision for cesarean section	42

Care after birth

Keeping newborn babies warm	44
Prophylactic vitamin K to the baby to prevent hemorrhagic disease of the newborn	44
Nasopharyngeal suctioning of infants who have passed meconium before birth	44
Presence of someone skilled in neonatal resuscitation at birth of all infants likely to be at risk	44
Oxygen for resuscitation of distressed newborn infants	44
Cardiac massage for infants born with absent heart beat	44
Naloxone for infants with respiratory depression due to narcotic administration before birth	44
Encouraging early mother-infant contact	45
Allowing mothers access to their own supply of symptom-relieving drugs in hospital	45
Consistent advice to new mothers	45
Offering choice in the length of hospital stay after childbirth	45
Telephone service of advice and information after women go home from hospital after birth	45
Psychological support for women depressed after childbirth	45
Encouraging early breastfeeding when mother and baby are ready	46
Skilled help with first breastfeed	46
Flexibility in breastfeeding practices	46
Antibiotics for infectious mastitis in breastfeeding women	46
Breast binding and fluid restriction for suppression of lactation	48
Support and care programs for bereaved parents	49
Encouraging parental contact with a dying or dead baby	49
Providing parents with prompt, accurate information about a severely ill baby	49
Encouraging autopsy for a dead baby and discussing the results with the parents	49
Help with funeral arrangements for a dead baby	49
Self-help groups for bereaved parents	49

Table 3. Forms of Care with a Trade-off between Beneficial and Adverse Effects

Women and caregivers should weigh these effects according
to circumstances, priorities, and preferences — *Chapter*

Basic care

Continuity of caregiver for childbearing women	3
Legislation restricting type of employment for pregnant women	3

Screening and diagnosis

Formal systems of risk scoring	7
Routine ultrasound in early pregnancy	8
Chorionic villus sampling versus amniocentesis for diagnosis of chromosomal abnormalities	9
Serum alpha-fetoprotein screening for neural tube defects	9
Triple-test screening for Down syndrome and neural tube defects	9

Pregnancy problems

Corticosteroids to promote fetal maturity before preterm birth in diabetic pregnancy	20, 25
Routine elective cesarean for breech presentation	22
Induction of labor for prelabor rupture of the membranes at term	23
Oral betamimetics to maintain uterine quiescence after arrest of preterm labor	24
Cervical cerclage for women at risk of preterm birth	24
Betamimetic drugs to stop preterm labor	24
Induction instead of surveillance for pregnancy after 41 weeks gestation	26
Expectant care versus induction of labor after fetal death	27

Childbirth

Continuous electronic monitoring (with scalp sampling) versus intermittent auscultation during labor	30
Midline versus mediolateral episiotomy, when episiotomy is necessary	32
Prophylactic ergometrine/oxytocin (syntometrine) versus oxytocin alone in the third stage of labor	33

Problems during childbirth

Routine preloading with intravenous fluids before epidural analgesia	34
Narcotics to relieve pain in labor	34
Inhalation analgesia to relieve pain in labor	34
Epidural analgesia to relieve pain in labor	34
Epidural administration of opiates to relieve pain in labor	34
Early amniotomy in spontaneous labor	35

Techniques of induction and operative delivery

Mechanical methods for cervical ripening or induction of labor	39, 40
Endocervical versus vaginal prostaglandin for cervical ripening before induction of labor	39
Oral prostaglandin E_2 for induction of labor with a ripe cervix	40
Natural prostaglandins versus oxytocin for induction of labor	40
Soft versus rigid vacuum extractor cups	41
Regional versus general anesthesia for cesarean section	42
Epidural versus spinal anesthesia for cesarean section	42
Ampicillin versus broader spectrum antibiotics for cesarean section	43

Care after childbirth

Prophylactic antibiotic eye ointments to prevent eye infection in the newborn	44
Prophylactic versus "rescue" surfactant for very preterm infants	44

Table 4. Forms of Care of Unknown Effectiveness

There are insufficient or inadequate quality data upon which to base a recommendation for practice	*Chapter*
Basic care	
Formal preconceptional care for all women	5
Fish oil supplementation to improve pregnancy outcome	6, 15
Prostaglandin precursors to improve pregnancy outcome	6, 15
Calcium supplementation to improve pregnancy outcome	6, 15, 24
Magnesium supplementation to improve pregnancy outcome	6, 15, 24
Zinc supplementation to improve pregnancy outcome	6
Antigen-avoidance diets to reduce risk of an atopic child	6
Screening and diagnosis	
Placental grading by ultrasound to improve perinatal outcome	8, 12
Measuring placental proteins for pre-eclampsia	10
Doppler ultrasound of uterine artery for pre-eclampsia	10
Measuring hematocrit and platelets for following the course of pre-eclampsia	10
Fetal biophysical profile for fetal surveillance	12
Pregnancy problems	
Acupressure for nausea and vomiting of pregnancy if simple measures are ineffective	13
Vitamin B6 for nausea and vomiting of pregnancy if simple measures are ineffective	13
Ginger for nausea and vomiting of pregnancy	13
Acid-suppressing drugs for heartburn	13
Rutosides for hemorrhoids	13
Rutosides for varicose veins	13
Exercise and education programs for backache	13
Increased salt intake for leg cramps	13
Oral magnesium for leg cramps	13
Progestogens for threatened miscarriage with a live fetus	14
Human chorionic gonadotrophin (HCG) for threatened miscarriage with a live fetus	14
Steroids for women with auto-antibodies and recurrent miscarriage	14
Evacuation versus "wait and see" following spontaneous miscarriage	14
Medical versus surgical evacuation following spontaneous miscarriage	14
Hospitalization for women with pregnancy-induced hypertension	15
Bed-rest for women with pre-eclampsia	15
Antihypertensive drugs for mild to moderate hypertension	15
Antioxidant vitamins C and E to prevent pre-eclampsia	15
Magnesium sulphate for pre-eclampsia	15
Interventionist versus expectant management for severe early onset pre-eclampsia	15
Plasma volume expansion for pre-eclampsia	15
Hospitalization and bed-rest for impaired fetal growth	16
Abdominal decompression for impaired fetal growth	16
Betamimetics for impaired fetal growth	16
Oxygen treatment for impaired fetal growth	16
Hormone treatment for impaired fetal growth	16
Calcium channel blockers for impaired fetal growth	16
Plasma volume expanders for impaired fetal growth	16
Hospitalization and bed-rest for triplet and higher order pregnancy	17
Antiviral agents for women with a history of recurrent genital herpes	19
Prophylactic antibiotics for prelabor rupture of membranes at term or preterm	23
Postpartum prophylactic antibiotics after prelabor rupture of membranes	23
Bed-rest to prevent preterm birth	24
Progestogens to prevent preterm birth	24
Calcium antagonists to stop preterm labor	24
Antibiotic treatment in preterm labor	24
Oxytocin antagonists to stop preterm labor	24

Table 4. Continued

There are insufficient or inadequate quality data upon which to base a recommendation for practice	*Chapter*
Sweeping of the membranes to prevent post-term pregnancy	26, 40
Nipple stimulation to prevent post-term pregnancy	26

Childbirth

Pre-admission assessment to determine if labor is in the active phase	29
Routine amnioscopy to detect meconium-stained amniotic fluid in labor	30
Routine artificial rupture of the membranes to detect meconium-stained amniotic fluid in labor	30
Short periods of electronic fetal monitoring as a screening test on admission in labor	30
Fetal stimulation tests for fetal assessment in labor	30
Maternal oxygen administration for fetal distress in labor	30
Institutional routines for repeating blood pressure measurements in labor	31
Nipple stimulation to prevent postpartum hemorrhage	33
Misoprostol in the third stage of labor to prevent postpartum hemorrhage	33
Early versus late clamping of the umbilical cord at birth	33
Methods for delivery of the placenta in the third stage of labor	33
Injecting oxytocin in the umbilical vein in the third stage of labor	33
Injecting oxytocin in the umbilical vein for retained placenta	33

Problems during childbirth

Abdominal decompression to relieve pain in labor	34
Immersion in water to relieve pain in labor	34
Acupuncture to relieve pain in labor	34
Acupressure to relieve pain in labor	34
Transcutaneous electrical nerve stimulation to relieve pain in labor	34
Intradermal injection of sterile water to relieve pain in labor	34
Aromatherapy to relieve pain in labor	34
Hypnosis to relieve pain in labor	34
Continuous infusion versus intermittent top-ups for epidural analgesia	34
Free mobility during labor to augment slow labor	35
Early use of oxytocin to augment slow or prolonged labor	35
"Active management" of labor	35
Cervical vibration for slow or prolonged labor	35
Histoacryl tissue adhesive for perineal skin repair	36
Cesarean section for very preterm delivery	37
Cesarean section for preterm breech delivery	37
Immediate versus delayed clamping of the umbilical cord of preterm infants	37

Techniques of induction and operative delivery

Oxytocin by automatic-infusion systems versus "standard regimens" for induction of labor	40
Misoprostol orally or vaginally for induction of labor	40
Use of hemostatic stapler for the uterine incision at cesarean section	42
Single-versus two-layer closure of the uterine incision at cesarean section	42
Systemic versus intraperitoneal prophylactic antibiotics at cesarean section	43

Care after childbirth

Tracheal suctioning for meconium in babies without respiratory depression	44
Routine use of antiseptics on the umbilical cord stump	45
Oral proteolytic enzymes for breast engorgement in breastfeeding mothers	46
Cabbage leaves for breast engorgement in breastfeeding mothers	46
Dopamine agonists to improve milk supply in breastfeeding mothers	46
Oxytocin nasal spray to improve milk supply in breastfeeding mothers	46
Oral proteolytic enzymes for perineal pain postpartum	47
Ultrasound and pulsed electromagnetic energy for perineal pain	47
Rubber rings and similar devices to prevent pressure for perineal pain	47
Cabergoline versus physical methods of suppressing lactation	48

Table 5. Forms of Care Unlikely to Be Beneficial

The evidence against these forms of care is not as firmly established as for those in Table 6	*Chapter*
Basic care	
Reliance on expert opinion instead of on good evidence for decisions about care	2
Routinely involving doctors in the care of all women during pregnancy and childbirth	3
Routinely involving obstetricians in the care of all women during pregnancy and childbirth	3
Not involving obstetricians in the care of women with serious risk factors	3
Fragmentation of care during pregnancy and childbirth	3
Social support for high-risk women to prevent preterm birth	3, 24
Antenatal breast or nipple care for women who plan to breastfeed	46
Advice to restrict sexual activity during pregnancy	5
Prohibition of all alcohol intake during pregnancy	5
Imposing dietary restrictions during pregnancy	6
Routine vitamin supplementation in late pregnancy in well-nourished populations	6
Routine hematinic supplementation in pregnancy in well-nourished populations	6
High-protein dietary supplementation	6, 16
Restriction of salt intake to prevent pre-eclampsia	6, 15
Screening and diagnosis	
Routine use of ultrasound for fetal measurement in late pregnancy	8, 12
Reliance on edema to screen for pre-eclampsia	10
Angiotensin-sensitivity test to screen for pre-eclampsia	10
Cold-pressor test to screen for pre-eclampsia	10
Roll-over test to screen for pre-eclampsia	10
Isometric exercise test to screen for pre-eclampsia	10
Measuring uric acid as a diagnostic test for pre-eclampsia	10
Screening for "gestational diabetes"	11
Routine glucose challenge test during pregnancy	11
Routine measurement of blood glucose during pregnancy	11
Insulin plus diet treatment for "gestational diabetes"	11
Diet treatment for "gestational diabetes"	11
Routine fetal movement counting to improve perinatal outcome	12
Routine use of Doppler ultrasound screening in all pregnancies	12
Measurement of placental proteins or hormones (including estriol and human placental lactogen)	12
Routine cervical assessment for prevention of preterm birth	24
Pregnancy problems	
Calcium supplementation for leg cramps	13
Screening for, and treatment of, vaginal candidal colonization without symptoms	13
Screening for, and treatment of, vaginal trichomonas colonization without symptoms	13
Screening for, and treatment of, bacterial vaginosis without symptoms	13
Bed-rest for threatened miscarriage	14
Immunotherapy for recurrent miscarriage	14
Antithrombotic agents to prevent pre-eclampsia	15
Reducing salt intake to prevent pre-eclampsia	15
Diazoxide for pre-eclampsia or hypertension in pregnancy	15
Ketanserin for severe hypertension in pregnancy	15
Diuretics for pregnancy-induced hypertension	15
High protein dietary supplementation for impaired fetal growth	16
Hospitalization and bed-rest for uncomplicated twin pregnancy	17
Cervical cerclage for multiple pregnancy	17
Prophylactic betamimetics for multiple pregnancy	17
Routine cesarean section for multiple pregnancy	17

Table 5. Continued

The evidence against these forms of care is not as firmly established as for those in Table 6	*Chapter*
Routine screening for mycoplasmas during pregnancy	19
Screening for toxoplasmosis during pregnancy	19
Treatment of group B streptococcus colonization during pregnancy	19
Cesarean section for non-active herpes simplex before or at the onset of labor	19
Amniotomy in HIV-infected women	19, 35
Elective delivery before term in women with otherwise uncomplicated diabetes	20
Elective cesarean section for pregnant women with diabetes	20
Discouraging breastfeeding in women with diabetes	20
Vaginal or rectal examination when placenta previa is suspected	21
Postural techniques for turning breech into cephalic presentation	22
External cephalic version before term to avoid breech presentation at birth	22
X-ray pelvimetry to diagnose cephalopelvic disproportion	22
Computer tomographic pelvimetry to predict cephalopelvic disproportion	22
Cesarean section for macrosomia without a trial of labor to prevent shoulder dystocia	22
Induction of labor to prevent cephalopelvic disproportion	22
Amniocentesis for prelabor rupture of the membranes preterm	23
Prophylactic tocolytics with prelabor rupture of the membranes preterm	23
Regular leucocyte counts for surveillance in prelabor rupture of the membranes	23
Home uterine activity monitoring for prevention of preterm birth	24
Magnesium sulphate to stop preterm labor	24
Betamimetics for preterm labor in women with heart disease or diabetes	24
Hydration to arrest preterm labor	24
Diazoxide to stop preterm labor	24
Adding thyrotrophin releasing hormone (TRH) to corticosteroids to promote fetal maturation	25
Childbirth	
Withholding food and drink from women in labor	29
Routine intravenous infusion in labor	29
Routine measurement of intrauterine pressure during oxytocin administration	31, 35
Wearing face masks during labor or for vaginal examinations	31
Frequent scheduled vaginal examinations in labor	31
Routine directed pushing during the second stage of labor	32
Pushing by sustained bearing down during the second stage of labor	32
Breath holding during the second stage of labor	32
Early bearing down during the second stage of labor	32
Arbitrary limitation of the duration of the second stage of labor	32
"Ironing out" or massaging the perineum during the second stage of labor	32
Routine manual exploration of the uterus after vaginal birth	32
Injectable prostaglandins in the third stage of labor	33
Encouraging early suckling to prevent postpartum hemorrhage	33
Problems during childbirth	
Injecting saline into the umbilical vein for retained placenta	33
Biofeedback to relieve pain in labor	34
Sedatives and tranquilizers to relieve pain in labor	34
Caudal block to relieve pain in labor	34
Paracervical block to relieve pain in labor	34
Intrapartum x-ray to diagnose cephalopelvic disproportion	35
Diagnosing cephalopelvic disproportion without ensuring adequate uterine contractions	35
Relaxin for slow or prolonged labor	35

Table 5. Continued

The evidence against these forms of care is not
as firmly established as for those in Table 6   *Chapter*

Hyaluronidase for slow or prolonged labor   35
Vitamin K to the mother to prevent intraventricular hemorrhage in the very preterm infant   37
Phenobarbitone to the mother to prevent intraventricular hemorrhage in the very preterm infant   37
Delivery of a very preterm infant without adequate facilities to care for a very preterm baby   37
Elective forceps delivery for preterm birth   37, 41
Routine use of episiotomy for preterm birth   37
Trial of labor after previous classical cesarean section   38
Routine manual exploration of the uterus to assess a previous cesarean section scar   38

Techniques of induction and operative delivery
Relaxin for cervical ripening before induction of labor   39
Nipple stimulation for cervical ripening before induction of labor   39
Extra-amniotic instead of other prostaglandin regimens for cervical ripening   39
Instrumental vaginal delivery to shorten the second stage of labor   41
Routine exteriorization of the uterus for repair of the uterine incision at cesarean section 42

Care after childbirth
Silver nitrate to prevent eye infection in newborn babies   44
Elective tracheal intubation for very low-birthweight infants who are not depressed   44
Routine suctioning of newborn babies   44
Medicated bathing of babies to reduce infection   45
Wearing hospital gowns in newborn nurseries   45
Restricting sibling visits to babies in hospital   45
Routine measurements of temperature, pulse, blood pressure, and fundal height postpartum   45
Limiting use of women's own non-prescription drugs postpartum in hospital   45
Administering non-prescription symptom-relieving drugs at regularly set intervals   45
Prohibition of oral contraceptives for diabetic women   20
Nipple shields for breastfeeding mothers   46
Switching breasts before babies spontaneously terminate the feed   46
Oxytocin for breast engorgement in breastfeeding mothers   46
Antibiotics for localized breast engorgement (milk stasis)   46
Discontinuing breastfeeding for localized breast engorgement (milk stasis)   46
Combinations of local anesthetics and topical steroids for relief of perineal pain   47
Relying on these tables without referring to the rest of the book   50

Table 6. Forms of Care Likely to Be Ineffective or Harmful

Ineffectiveness or harm demonstrated by clear evidence	Chapter
Basic care	
Dietary restriction to prevent pre-eclampsia	6, 15
Screening and diagnosis	
Contraction stress cardiotocography to improve perinatal outcome	12
Nipple-simulation test cardiotocography to improve perinatal outcome	12
Non-selective use of non-stress cardiotocography to improve perinatal outcome	12
Pregnancy problems	
Adrenocorticotrophic hormone (ACTH) for severe vomiting of pregnancy	13
Saline cathartics for constipation	13
Lubricant oils for constipation	13
Diethylstilbestrol during pregnancy	14
Elective delivery for prelabor rupture of the membranes preterm	23
Ethanol to stop preterm labor	24
Progestogens to stop preterm labor	24
Childbirth	
Routine enema in labor	29
Routine pubic shaving in preparation for childbirth	29
Electronic fetal monitoring without access to fetal scalp sampling during labor	30
Prophylactic intrapartum amnio-infusion for oligohydramnios	30
Rectal examinations to assess labor progress	31
Requiring a supine (flat on back) position in the second stage of labor	32
Routine use of the lithotomy position for the second stage of labor	32
Routine or liberal episiotomy for birth	32
Ergometrine instead of oxytocin prophylaxis in the third stage of labor	33
Problems in childbirth	
Glycerol-impregnated catgut for repair of perineal trauma	36
Techniques of induction and operative delivery	
Oral prostaglandins for cervical ripening	39
Estrogens for cervical ripening or for induction of labor	39
Oxytocin for cervical ripening before induction of labor	39
Care after childbirth	
Sodium bicarbonate for asphyxiated babies	44
Routine restriction of mother-infant contact	45
Routine nursery care for babies in hospital	45
Antenatal Hoffman's exercises for inverted or flat nipples	46
Antenatal breast shells for inverted or flat nipples	46
Limitation of suckling time during breastfeeding	46
Nipple creams or ointments for breastfeeding mothers	46
Routine supplements of water or formula for breastfed babies	46
Samples of formula for breastfeeding mothers	46
Encouraging fluid intake beyond demands of thirst for breastfeeding mothers	46
Combined estrogen-progesterone oral contraceptives for breastfeeding mothers	46
Test weighing of breastfed infants	46
Witchhazel for relief of perineal pain	47
Adding salt to bath water for treating perineal pain	47
Antiseptic solutions added to bath water for perineal pain	47
Hormones for relief of breast symptoms in non-breastfeeding mothers	48
Bromocriptine for relief of breast symptoms in non-breastfeeding mothers	48

Murray Enkin is Professor Emeritus, Departments of Obstetrics and Gynecology, Clinical Epidemiology and Biostatistics, McMaster University, Hamilton, Ontario, Canada; Marc Keirse is Professor and Head, Department of Obstetrics, Gynaecology and Reproductive Medicine, The Flinders University of South Australia, Adelaide, South Australia; James Neilson is Professor of Obstetrics and Gynaecology, University of Liverpool, Liverpool, United Kingdom; Caroline Crowther is Associate Professor, Department of Obstetrics and Gynaecology, University of Adelaide, Adelaide, South Australia; Lelia Duley is Obstetric Epidemiologist, Institute of Health Sciences, Oxford, United Kingdom; Ellen Hodnett is Professor and Heather M. Reisman Chair in Perinatal Nursing Research, University of Toronto, Toronto, Ontario, Canada; and Justus Hofmeyr is Professor of Obstetrics and Gynaecology, Coronation Hospital and University of the Witwatersrand, Johannesburg, South Africa.

Reprinted by permission of the authors.

THE MOTHER-FRIENDLY CHILDBIRTH INITIATIVE

THE FIRST CONSENSUS INITIATIVE OF THE COALITION FOR IMPROVING MATERNITY SERVICES

Mission

The Coalition for Improving Maternity Services (CIMS) is a coalition of individuals and national organizations with concern for the care and well-being of mothers, babies, and families. Our mission is to promote a wellness model of maternity care that will improve birth outcomes and substantially reduce costs. This evidence-based mother-, baby-, and family-friendly model focuses on prevention and wellness as the alternatives to high-cost screening, diagnosis, and treatment programs.

> ***Glossary**
> - *birth center:* Free-standing maternity center
> - *doula:* A woman who gives continuous physical, emotional, and informational support during labor and birth—may also provide postpartum care in the home.
> - *episiotomy:* Surgically cutting to widen the vaginal opening for birth.
> - *induction:* Artificially starting labor.
> - *morbidity:* Disease or injury.
> - *perinatal:* Around the time of birth.
> - *rupture of membranes:* Breaking the "bag of waters."

Preamble

Whereas:

- In spite of spending far more money per capita on maternity and newborn care than any other country, the United States falls behind most industrialized countries in perinatal* morbidity* and mortality, and maternal mortality is four times greater for African-American women than for Euro-American women;
- Midwives attend the vast majority of births in those industrialized countries with the best perinatal outcomes, yet in the United States, midwives are the principal attendants at only a small percentage of births;
- Current maternity and newborn practices that contribute to high costs and inferior outcomes include the inappropriate application of technology and routine procedures that are not based on scientific evidence;

- Increased dependence on technology has diminished confidence in women's innate ability to give birth without intervention;
- The integrity of the mother-child relationship, which begins in pregnancy, is compromised by the obstetrical treatment of mother and baby as if they were separate units with conflicting needs;
- Although breastfeeding has been scientifically shown to provide optimum health, nutritional, and developmental benefits to newborns and their mothers, only a fraction of U.S. mothers are fully breastfeeding their babies by the age of six weeks;
- The current maternity care system in the United States does not provide equal access to health care resources for women from disadvantaged population groups, women without insurance, and women whose insurance dictates caregivers or place of birth;

Therefore,

We, the undersigned members of CIMS, hereby resolve to define and promote mother-friendly maternity services in accordance with the following principles:

Principles

We believe the philosophical cornerstones of mother-friendly care to be as follows:

Normalcy of the Birthing Process

- Birth is a normal, natural, and healthy process.
- Women and babies have the inherent wisdom necessary for birth.
- Babies are aware, sensitive human beings at the time of birth, and should be acknowledged and treated as such.
- Breastfeeding provides the optimum nourishment for newborns and infants.
- Birth can safely take place in hospitals, birth centers, and homes.
- The midwifery model of care, which supports and protects the normal birth process, is the most appropriate for the majority of women during pregnancy and birth.

Empowerment

- A woman's confidence and ability to give birth and to care for her baby are enhanced or diminished by every person who gives her care, and by the environment in which she gives birth.
- A mother and baby are distinct yet interdependent during pregnancy, birth, and infancy. Their interconnectedness is vital and must be respected.
- Pregnancy, birth, and the postpartum period are milestone events in the continuum of life. These experiences profoundly affect women, babies, fathers, and families, and have important and long-lasting effects on society.

Autonomy

Every woman should have the opportunity to:
- Have a healthy and joyous birth experience for herself and her family, regardless of her age or circumstances;
- Give birth as she wishes in an environment in which she feels nurtured and secure, and her emotional well-being, privacy, and personal preferences are respected;
- Have access to the full range of options for pregnancy, birth, and nurturing her baby, and to accurate information on all available birthing sites, caregivers, and practices;
- Receive accurate and up-to-date information about the benefits and risks of all procedures, drugs, and tests suggested for use during pregnancy, birth, and the postpartum period, with the rights to informed consent and informed refusal;
- Receive support for making informed choices about what is best for her and her baby based on her individual values and beliefs.

Do No Harm

- Interventions should not be applied routinely during pregnancy, birth, or the postpartum period. Many standard medical tests, procedures, technologies, and drugs carry risks to both mother and baby, and should be avoided in the absence of specific scientific indications for their use.
- If complications arise during pregnancy, birth, or the postpartum period, medical treatments should be evidence-based.

Responsibility

- Each caregiver is responsible for the quality of care she or he provides.
- Maternity care practice should be based not on the needs of the caregiver or provider, but solely on the needs of the mother and child.
- Each hospital and birth center is responsible for the periodic review and evaluation, according to current scientific evidence, of the effectiveness, risks, and rates of use of its medical procedures for mothers and babies.
- Society, through both its government and the public health establishment, is responsible for ensuring access to maternity services for all women, and for monitoring the quality of those services.
- Individuals are ultimately responsible for making informed choices about the health care they and their babies receive.

These principles give rise to the following steps which support, protect, and promote mother-friendly maternity services:

TEN STEPS OF THE MOTHER-FRIENDLY CHILDBIRTH INITIATIVE

For Mother-Friendly Hospitals, Birth Centers,* and Home Birth Services

To receive CIMS designation as Mother-Friendly, a hospital, birth center, or home birth service must carry out the above philosophical principles by fulfilling the Ten Steps of Mother-Friendly Care:

A mother-friendly hospital, birth center, or home birth service:
1. Offers all birthing mothers:
   - Unrestricted access to the birth companions of her choice, including fathers, partners, children, family members, and friends;
   - Unrestricted access to continuous emotional and physical support from a skilled woman—for example, a doula* or labor-support professional;

- Access to professional midwifery care.

2. Provides accurate descriptive and statistical information to the public about its practices and procedures for birth care, including measures of interventions and outcomes.

3. Provides culturally competent care—that is, care that is sensitive and responsive to the specific beliefs, values, and customs of the mother's ethnicity and religion.

4. Provides the birthing woman with the freedom to walk, move about, and assume the positions of her choice during labor and birth (unless restriction is specifically required to correct a complication), and discourages the use of the lithotomy (flat on back with legs elevated) position.

5. Has clearly defined policies and procedures for:
   - collaborating and consulting throughout the perinatal period with other maternity services, including communicating with the original caregiver when transfer from one birth site to another is necessary;
   - linking the mother and baby to appropriate community resources, including prenatal and postdischarge follow-up and breastfeeding support.

6. Does not routinely employ practices and procedures that are unsupported by scientific evidence, including but not limited to the following:
   - shaving;
   - enemas;
   - IVs (intravenous drip);
   - withholding nourishment or water;
   - early rupture of membranes*;
   - electronic fetal monitoring.

Other interventions are limited as follows:
- Has an induction* rate of 10% or less;
- Has an episiotomy* rate of 20% or less, with a goal of 5% or less;
- Has a total cesarean rate of 10% or less in community hospitals, and 15% or less in tertiary care (high-risk) hospitals;
- Has a VBAC (vaginal birth after cesarean) rate of 60% or more with a goal of 75% or more.

7. Educates staff in non-drug methods of pain relief, and does not promote the use of analgesic or anesthetic drugs not specifically required to correct a complication.
8. Encourages all mothers and families, including those with sick or premature newborns or infants with congenital problems, to touch, hold, breastfeed, and care for their babies to the extent compatible with their conditions.
9. Discourages non-religious circumcision of the newborn.
10. Strives to achieve the WHO-UNICEF "Ten Steps of the Baby-Friendly Hospital Initiative" to promote successful breastfeeding:
    1. *Have a written breastfeeding policy that is routinely communicated to all health care staff;*
    2. *Train all health care staff in skills necessary to implement this policy;*
    3. *Inform all pregnant women about the benefits and management of breastfeeding;*
    4. *Help mothers initiate breastfeeding within a half-hour of birth;*
    5. *Show mothers how to breastfeed and how to maintain lactation even if they should be separated from their infants;*
    6. *Give newborn infants no food or drink other than breast milk unless medically indicated;*
    7. *Practice rooming in: allow mothers and infants to remain together 24 hours a day;*
    8. *Encourage breastfeeding on demand;*
    9. *Give no artificial teat or pacifiers (also called dummies or soothers) to breastfeeding infants;*
    10. *Foster the establishment of breastfeeding support groups and refer mothers to them on discharge from hospitals or clinics.*

Bibliography

American College of Obstetricians and Gynecologists. Fetal heart rate patterns: monitoring, interpretation, and management. *Technical Bulletin* No. 207, July 1995.

—. Guidelines for vaginal delivery after a previous cesarean birth. *ACOG Committee Opinion* 1988; No 64.

Canadian Paediatric Soc, Fetus, and Newborn Committee. Neonatal circumcision revisited. *Can Med Assoc J* 1996;154(6):769-780.

Enkin M, et al. *A Guide to Effective Care in Pregnancy and Childbirth* 2nd rev ed. Oxford: Oxford University Press, 1995. (Data from this book come from the Cochrane Database of Perinatal Trials.)

Goer H. *Obstetric Myths Versus Research Realities: A Guide to the Medical Literature.* Westport, CT: Bergin and Garvey, 1995.

Bureau of Maternal and Child Health. Unity through diversity: a report on the Healthy Mothers Healthy Babies Coalition Communities of Color Leadership Roundtable. Healthy Mothers Healthy Babies, 1993. (A copy may obtained by calling (202) 821-8993 ext. 254. Dr. Marsden Wagner also provided maternal mortality statistics from official state health data.)

International Lactation Consultant Association. Position paper on infant feeding. rev 1994. Chicago: ILCA, 1994.

Klaus M, Kennell JH, and Klaus PH. *Mothering the Mother.* Menlo Park, CA: Addison-Wesley, 1993.

—. *Bonding: Building the Foundations of Secure Attachment and Independence.* Menlo Park, CA: Addison-Wesley, 1995.

Wagner M. *Pursuing the Birth Machine: The Search for Appropriate Birth Technology.* Australia: ACE Graphics, 1994. (Dr. Wagner's book has the "General Recommendations" of *The WHO* Fortaleza, Brazil, April, 1985 and the "Summary Report" of *The WHO Consensus Conference on Appropriate Technology Following Birth* Trieste, October, 1986.)

Ratified by these members of the Coalition for Improving Maternity Services (CIMS), July, 1996

Organizations

(Names of organizations' officers may have changed since ratification.)

Academy of Certified Birth Educators (Olathe, KS), Linda M. Herrick, RNC, BSN, CCE, CD; and Sally Riley, BSEd, CCE, CD, & Judie C. Wika, RNC, MSN, CNM, CCE, Co-Directors

American Academy of Husband-Coached Childbirth (The Bradley Method™), (Sherman Oaks, CA), Jay and Marjie Hathaway, Executive Directors

American College of Nurse-Midwives (Washington, DC), Joyce Roberts, CNM, PhD, FACNM, President

American College of Domiciliary Midwives (Palo Alto, CA), Faith Gibson, CPM, Executive Director

Association of Labor Assistants and Childbirth Educators (Cambridge, MA), Jessica L. Porter, President

Association for Pre- & Perinatal Psychology and Health (Geyserville, CA), David B. Chamberlain, PhD, President

Association of Women's Health, Obstetric, and Neonatal Nurses (Washington, DC), Joy Grohar, RNC, MS, President

Attachment Parenting International, (Nashville, TN), Lysa Parker, BS, & Barbara Nicholson, MEd, Co-Founders

Birthworks, Inc. (Medford, NJ), Cathy E. W. Daub, RPT, CCE, President

Center for Perinatal Research & Family Support (River Vale, NJ), Debra Pascali-Bonaro, Executive Director

Doulas of North America (Seattle, WA), Barbara A. Hotelling, RN, BSN, CD, FACCE, President
The Farm (Summertown, TN), Ina May Gaskin, President
Global Maternal/Child Health Association (Wilsonville, OR), Barbara Harper, RN, President
Informed Home Birth/Informed Birth & Parenting (Fair Oaks, CA), Rahima Baldwin
    Dancy, CPM, President
International Association of Infant Massage (Oak View, CA), Ellen Kerr, RN, BSN, MST,
    CIMI, President
International Childbirth Education Association (Minneapolis, MN), Cheryl Coleman, RN,
    BSN, ICCE, President
International Lactation Consultant Association (Raleigh, NC), Karen Kerkhoff Gromada,
    MSN, RN, IBCLC, President
La Leche League International (Schaumburg, IL), Carol Kolar, RN, Director of Education
    & Outreach
Lamaze International (formerly ASPO/Lamaze), (Washington, DC), Deborah Woolley,
    CNM, PhD, FACCE, President
Midwifery Today (Eugene, OR), Jan Tritten, TMME, Editor
Midwives Alliance of North America (Newton, KS), Ina May Gaskin, President
Midwives of Santa Cruz (Santa Cruz, CA), Roxanne Potter, CNM, Kate Bowland, CNM,
    Co-Directors
National Association of Childbearing Centers (Perkiomenville, PA), Susan Stapleton, MSN,
    CNM, President
National Association of Postpartum Care Services (Denver, CO), Gerri Levrini, RN, MSN,
    CNAA, President
North American Registry of Midwives (Nashville, TN), Sharon Wells, MS, LM,CPM,
    Coordinator
Wellness Assoc. (Ashville, NC), John W. Travis, MD, MPH, & Meryn G. Callander, ME,
    BSW, Co-Directors

Individuals
Sondra Abdulla-Zaimah, RN, CNM, CPM, Senegal, W. Africa
Shannon Anton, CPM, San Francisco, CA
Susanne Arms, Bayfield, CO, *Immaculate Deception*
Gini Baker, RN, MPH, IBCLC, FACCE, Escondido, CA
Maggie Bennett, LM, CPM, Seaside, CA
Brian Berman, Bainbridge Island, WA
Mary Brucker, CNM, DNSc, Dallas, TX
Raymond Castellino, DC, RPP, Santa Barbara, CA
Elena Carrillo, LCCE, FACCE, CD, Mexico City, Mexico
Robbie Davis-Floyd, PhD, Austin, TX, *Birth as an American Rite of Passage*
Henci Goer, ACCE, Sunnyvale, CA, *The Thinking Woman's Guide to a Better Birth*
Dorothy Harrison, IBCLC, Edmunds WA
Jack Heinowitz, PhD, San Diego, CA, *Pregnant Fathers*
Tina Kimmel, MSW, MPH, Berkeley, CA
Marshall Klaus, MD, Berkeley, CA, *Bonding—Building the Foundation for Secure
    Attachment and Independence*
Phyllis Klaus, CSW, MFCC, Berkeley, CA, *The Amazing Newborn*
Judith Lothian, RN, PhD, FACC, Brooklyn, NY
Susan Sobin Pease, MBA, CIMI, CMT, San Francisco, CA
Paulina G. Perez, RN, BSN, FACCE, Johnson, VT *Special Women*
James W. Prescott, PhD, San Diego, CA, *Brain Function and Malnutrition*
Mayri Sagady, RN, CNM, MSN, San Diego, CA
Karen N. Salt, CCE, Coconino Community College, Flagstaff, AZ
Irene Sandvold, DrPH, CNM, Rockville, MD
Roberta M. Scaer, MSS, Boulder, CO, *A Good Birth, A Safe Birth*
Betsy K. Schwartz, MMHS, Coconut Creek, FL

Penny Simkin, PT, Seattle, WA, *Pregnancy, Childbirth, and the Newborn*
Linda J. Smith, BSE, FACCE, Bright Future Lactation Resource Ctr., Dayton, OH
Suzanne Suarez, JD, RN, Tampa, FL
Sandy Szalay, ARNP, CCE, Seattle, WA
Marsden Wagner, MD, MSPH, Washington, DC, *Pursuing the Birth Machine*
Diony Young, Geneseo, NY

A partial list of organizations and individuals endorsing this Initiative
(for current list, see www.motherfriendly.org)

Organizations
Academy for Guided Imagery, Mill Valley, CA
American Holistic Nurses Association
Birth Network of Santa Cruz County, CA
The Boston Women's Health Book Collective, Boston, MA
C/Sec, Inc., Ocean City, NJ
Canadian Society for the Prevention of Cruelty to Children, Midland, Ontario
Citizens for Midwifery, Athens, GA
The Compleat Mother, Minot, ND
Doctors Opposing Circumcision, Seattle, WA
International Cesarean Awareness Network, Redondo Beach, CA
The Massachusetts Friends of Midwives, Boston, MA
Mothering Magazine, Santa Fe, NM
National Association of Parents and Professionals for Safe Alternatives in Childbirth,
    Marble Hill, MO
National Center for Violence Prevention, Ashland, OR
The Nurturing Parent Journal Online, Prescott, AZ
Nurses for the Rights of the Child, Santa Fe, NM
Physicians for Midwifery, Lafayette, LA
Touch the Future, Nevada City, CA

Individuals
Patch Adams, MD, *Geshundeit!*
Thomas Armstrong, PhD, *The Radiant Child*
Elizabeth N. Baldwin, JD, North Miami Beach, FL
Elisabeth Bing, RPT, FACCE, *Six Practical Lessons for an Easy Childbirth*
David Bresler, PhD, Associate Clinical Professor of Anesthesiology, UCLA School of Medicine
Elliott E. Dacher, MD, *Whole Healing*
Rae Davies, BSH, The Birth Company
Larry Dossey, MD, *Prayer is Good Medicine*
Murray W. Enkin, MD, FRCS(C), Prof. Emeritus, Depts of Ob/Gyn, Clin. Epid., &
    Biostatistics, McMaster Univ., *A Guide to Effective Care in Pregnancy and Childbirth*
Eunice K. M. Ernst, CNM, MPH, Mary Breckinridge Chair of Midwifery Perkiomenville, PA
Sharron S. Humenick, PhD, RN, FAAN, Editor, *Journal of Perinatal Education*
Laura Huxley, *Children Are Our Ultimate Investment*
Dorothy J. Jongeward, PhD, *Born to Win*
Risa Kaparo, PhD, California Inst. of Integral Studies
John H. Kennell, MD, *Mothering the Mother*
George Leonard, *Mastery*
Jean Liedloff, *The Continuum Concept*
Ashley Montagu, PhD, *Touching*
Michel Odent, MD, *Birth Reborn*

Kathy Oriel, MD, Asst. Prof, Dept Family Medicine, U. of Wisc, Madison
Jeffery J. Patterson, DO, Prof, Dept Family Medicine, U. of Wisc, Madison
Joseph Chilton Pearce, *Magical Child*
Kent Peterson, MD, *Handbook of Health Assessment Tools*
Jane Pincus, *Our Bodies, Ourselves*
Judith Rooks, CNM, MPH, MS, FACNM, *Midwifery and Childbirth in America*
Martin F. Rubin, MD, Clinical Faculty, UC San Francisco, School of Medicine, Medical
    Director, Sonoma County (CA) Dept of Mental Health
Regina Sara Ryan, MA, *Wellness Workbook*
Linda J. Smith, BSE, FACCE, IBCLC, Bright Future Lactation Resource Centre
Patty Stuart-Macadam, PhD, Dept. Anthropology, U. of Toronto

Help Circulate this Initiative

CIMS (pronounced "kims") is a coalition of individuals and organizations volunteering their time to make childbirth a safer, more natural experience. Please help disseminate this Initiative by giving out copies, reprinting it in newsletters, sending it to local newspapers and government representatives, mentioning it on talk shows, etc. (with complete attribution). We urge you to mail copies (or forward the Web address) to appropriate friends and acquaintances along with a personal note requesting that they similarly forward it.

Get Free Copies of Our Publications

Copies of this document (as well as a simpler version for the general public—Having a Baby? Ten Questions to Ask) in both English and Spanish, can be downloaded at <www.motherfriendly.org>. Both are available in Acrobat Reader files (pdf) that print out compactly, as well as in "rich text format" (rtf) files that open in most word processors.

Get Paper Copies of Our Publications

For single copies send $3 ($4 Canada/Mexico, $5 all others) or in bulk: 25 copies/$10 ($12 Canada/Mexico, $15 all others); 100 copies/ $20 ($25 Canada/Mexico, $30 all others) to CIMS, PO Box 2346, Ponte Vedra Beach, FL 32004, US dollars only, prepayment required. (888) 282-CIMS, (904) 285-1613, Fax: (904) 285-2120.

Mother-Friendly Designation and the CIMS Discussion Forum

Help your local birth service achieve Mother-Friendly status via our self-assessment questionnaire available by mail or from <www.motherfriendly.org>. Join the online discussion forum through our Website to help support the dissemination and implementation of the Initiative. We also welcome comments and suggestions at the Website (if your comments are about the contents of the Initiative, please cite the relevant evidence-based material).

Appendix C
THE RIGHTS OF
CHILDBEARING WOMEN

The Maternity Center Association (MCA) is a not-for-profit organization that has been dedicated to improving maternity care in the United States since 1918. This statement outlines a set of basic rights that MCA has identified and promotes for all childbearing women. It applies widely accepted human rights to the specific situation of maternity care. Although most of these rights are granted to women in the United States by law, many women do not have knowledge of their rights.

Fundamental Problems with Maternity Care in the United States

This statement was developed in response to serious and continuing problems with maternity care in the United States, including:

- The United States is the only wealthy industrialized nation that does not guarantee access to essential health care for all pregnant women and infants. Many women, especially those with low incomes, lack access to adequate maternity care.
- A large body of scientific research shows that many widely used maternity care practices that involve risk and discomfort are of no benefit to low-risk women and infants. On the other hand, some practices that clearly offer important benefits are not widely available in U.S. hospitals.
- Many women do not receive adequate information about benefits and risks of specific procedures, drugs, tests, and treatments, or about alternatives.
- Childbearing women frequently are not aware of their legal right to make health care choices on behalf of themselves and their babies, and do not exercise this right.

We must ensure that all childbearing women have access to information and care that is based on the best scientific evidence now available, and that they understand and have opportunities to exercise their right to make health care decisions. Women whose rights are violated need access to legal or other recourse to address their grievances.

Every Woman's Rights

Consideration and respect for every woman under all circumstances is the foundation of this statement of rights.

1. Every woman has the right to health care before, during, and after pregnancy and childbirth.
2. Every woman and infant has the right to receive care that is consistent with current scientific evidence about benefits and risks.* Practices that have been found to be safe and beneficial should be used when indicated. Harmful, ineffective, or unnecessary practices should be avoided. Unproven interventions should be used only in the context of research to evaluate their effects.
3. Every woman has the right to choose a midwife or a physician as her maternity care provider. Both caregivers skilled in normal childbearing and caregivers skilled in complications are needed to ensure quality care for all.
4. Every woman has the right to choose her birth setting from the full range of safe options available in her community, on the basis of complete, objective information about benefits, risks and costs of these options.*
5. Every woman has the right to receive all or most of her maternity care from a single caregiver or a small group of caregivers, with whom she can establish a relationship. Every woman has the right to leave her maternity caregiver and select another if she becomes dissatisfied with her care.* (Only second sentence is a legal right.)
6. Every woman has the right to information about the professional identity and qualifications of those involved with her care, and to know when those involved are trainees.*
7. Every woman has the right to communicate with caregivers and receive all care in privacy, which may involve excluding nonessential personnel. She also has

the right to have all personal information treated according to standards of confidentiality.*

8. Every woman has the right to receive maternity care that identifies and addresses social and behavioral factors that affect her health and that of her baby.** She should receive information to help her take the best care of herself and her baby and have access to social services and behavioral change programs that could contribute to their health.

9. Every woman has the right to full and clear information about benefits, risks, and costs of the procedures, drugs, tests and treatments offered to her, and of all other reasonable options, including no intervention.* She should receive this information about all interventions that are likely to be offered during labor and birth well before the onset of labor.

10. Every woman has the right to accept or refuse procedures, drugs, tests and treatments, and to have her choices honored. She has the right to change her mind.* (Please note that this established legal right has been challenged in a number of recent cases.)

11. Every woman has the right to be informed if her caregivers wish to enroll her or her infant in a research study. She should receive full information about all known and possible benefits and risks of participation, and she has the right to decide whether to participate, free from coercion and without negative consequences.*

12. Every woman has the right to unrestricted access to all available records about her pregnancy, her labor, and her infant; to obtain a full copy of these records; and to receive help in understanding them, if necessary.*

13. Every woman has the right to receive maternity care that is appropriate to her cultural and religious background, and to receive information in a language in which she can communicate.*

14. Every woman has the right to have family members and friends of her choice present during all aspects of her maternity care.**

15. Every woman has the right to receive continuous social, emotional, and physical support during labor and birth

from a caregiver who has been trained in labor support.**

16. Every woman has the right to receive full advance information about risks and benefits of all reasonably available methods for relieving pain during labor and birth, including methods that do not require the use of drugs. She has the right to choose which methods will be used and to change her mind at any time.*

17. Every woman has the right to freedom of movement during labor, unencumbered by tubes, wires, or other apparatus. She also has the right to give birth in the position of her choice.*

18. Every woman has the right to virtually uninterrupted contact with her newborn from the moment of birth, as long as she and her baby are healthy and do not need care that requires separation.**

19. Every woman has the right to receive complete information about the benefits of breastfeeding well in advance of labor, to refuse supplemental bottles and other actions that interfere with breastfeeding, and to have access to skilled lactation support for as long as she chooses to breastfeed.**

20. Every woman has the right to decide collaboratively with caregivers when she and her baby will leave the birth site for home, based on their condition and circumstances.**

(At this time in the United States, childbearing women are legally entitled to those rights marked with *. The legal system would probably uphold those rights marked with **.)

© Maternity Center Association, 2004

Our Sources

The following sources have helped guide the development of this statement of rights:

1. American Hospital Association. A Patient's Bill of Rights, revised edition approved by the AHA Board of Trustees on October 21, 1992.
2. Annas, G. J. A national bill of patients' rights. New England Journal of Medicine 338, (10) 695-699, 1998.
3. Annas, G. J. The Rights of Patients, second edition. Carbondale, IL; Southern Illinois University Press, 1989.
4. Boston Women's Health Book Collective. Section on "Child-bearing" and chapter on "The politics of women's health and medical care." In: Our Bodies, Ourselves for the New Century. New York: Simon & Schuster, 1998, pp. 433-543, 680-722.
5. Coalition for Improving Maternity Services (CIMS). The Mother-Friendly Childbirth Initiative,1996. Available at: www.motherfriendly.org
6. Enkin, M., Keirse, M. J. N. C., Neilson, J., Crowther, C., Duley, L., Hodnett, E., and Hofmeyr, J. A Guide to Effective Care in Pregnancy and Childbirth, third edition. New York: Oxford University Press, 2000. Available at: www.maternitywise.org/guide/
7. International Childbirth Education Association, Inc. The Pregnant Patient's Bill of Rights. Minneapolis: ICEA, 1975.
8. President's Advisory Commission on Consumer Protection and Quality in the Health Care Industry. Appendix A: Consumer Bill of Rights and Responsibilities. In its Final Report: Quality First: Better Health Care for All Americans. Available at: www.hcqual-itycommission.gov/final/append_a.html
9. United Nations. Universal Declaration of Human Rights. Published by the United Nations, 1948.

The Maternity Center Association grants permission to any individual or organization to copy and distribute the Statement of Rights in its entirety as long as credit is given to the Maternity Center Association.

Thank you to George Annas, professor and chair of Health Law at the Boston University School of Public Health, for clarifying the legal status of the individual rights.

To Order a Printed Brochure:

For a single complimentary copy of *The Rights of Childbearing Women*, please send a self-addressed stamped envelope to: Maternity Center Association, 281 Park Avenue South, 5th Floor, New York, New York 10010. For multiple copies, consult www.maternitywise.org/bookstore/

Appendix D
Lamaze International Position Papers

Lamaze for the Twenty-First Century

Lamaze International is determined to get the word out that today's Lamaze is not the Lamaze of 1960. Forty years of research and learning from women's experience of normal, natural birth have provided evidence that has gradually but dramatically changed Lamaze from being a method for giving birth to a philosophy that provides the foundation and direction for women as they prepare to give birth and become mothers. "Breathing" is no longer the hallmark of Lamaze. The Lamaze Philosophy of Birth is at the heart of Lamaze education and has been for nearly a decade the driving force for significant changes in Lamaze preparation for childbirth. Today's Lamaze affirms the normalcy of birth, acknowledges women's inherent ability to birth their babies, and explores all the ways that women find strength and comfort during labor and birth.

Reframing Pain

Until recently, pain has been thought of as an unpleasant side effect of labor contractions. In Lamaze classes of the past, women only learned about the factors that influence pain perception and practiced techniques, including relaxation and breathing, that helped diminish the perception of pain. As our

---

Lamaze Philosophy of Birth

- Birth is normal, natural, and healthy.
- The experience of birth profoundly affects women and their families.
- Women's inner wisdom guides them through birth.
- Women's confidence and ability to give birth is either enhanced or diminished by the care provider and place of birth.
- Women have a right to give birth free from routine medical intervention.
- Birth can safely take place in homes, birth centers, and hospitals.
- Childbirth education empowers women to make informed choices in health care, to assume responsibility for their health, and to trust their inner wisdom.

understanding of normal labor and birth has evolved, we are beginning to have a better appreciation for the important role pain plays in the process of normal labor and birth. The pain of labor, like most pain, is protective. Responding to pain with movement, including walking, rocking, and position changes, not only helps the baby rotate and descend through the pelvis, but also protects a woman's body during the process. As the cervix stretches and dilates, oxytocin levels increase, and contractions strengthen and become more effective. As pain increases, endorphins are released that help women cope with the demands of the stronger contractions and the descent of the baby. Actively responding to the pain of contractions then not only promotes comfort but promotes the progress of labor. The Lamaze Certified Childbirth Educator encourages women to work actively with labor, finding comfort in response to what they are feeling.

Because the pain of labor is not associated with trauma, but is a part of a normal, physiologic process, it is sometimes compared to the pain associated with other challenging physical activities. Those who push themselves to climb the last hill, cross the finish line, or conquer a challenging dance routine often report feelings of euphoria and increased self-esteem. Researchers have found that women who experience natural birth often describe similar feelings of exaltation and increased self-esteem.[1] These feelings of accomplishment, confidence, and strength have the potential to transform women's lives. In many cultures, the runner who completes the long race is admired, but it is not acknowledged that the laboring woman may experience the same life-altering feelings. Lamaze helps each woman find ways to meet the challenges of birth confidently and purposefully, and to discover her strength in birth.

Rethinking Breathing and Relaxation

Relaxation and focusing on controlled breathing continue to be effective ways of decreasing pain perception, and are fairly simple comfort techniques to learn. But birth is active work, and finding comfort as labor progresses, for most women, requires more than focused attention and releasing tension. In today's Lamaze classes, women learn to respond to their contractions and find comfort in many ways including walking, rocking, position changes, massage, heat/cold therapy, hydrotherapy, slow dancing, and use of birth balls. These active comfort strategies are important because in providing comfort, they also promote the progress of labor.

Breathing is no longer taught or practiced to "get it right." Instead, women are taught that finding a breathing pattern is just one of a number of strategies that can be used to stay focused during contractions. Some women find that patterned breathing is a ritual, like prayer, rocking, or other behaviors done in a methodical way, that helps them move through contractions. Lamaze educators continue to teach body awareness and tension release, but the goal is not to expect total relaxation during labor. Rather, women are encouraged to be in the moment, not fearful, but actively relaxed, rhythmically working with labor.

Retiring the Coach

Lamaze classes emphasize the importance of continuous emotional and physical support in labor, but the "coach" who takes charge of the birth, calling the plays and instructing the mother, has been retired. Research suggests that when trained in class to take on the role of coach, few men actually do so.[2] More importantly, women know how to give birth; therefore encouragement and support, rather than "coaching," is required. In Lamaze classes, fathers and family learn how to provide quiet, gentle, encouraging support, and learn basic comfort measures that help most women in labor. Fathers and family learn that their calm, focused presence is the most important thing women need from them. Family members are encouraged to experience the birth of the baby in their own way. The role of the professional doula is discussed, and women who will give birth in a hospital environment that does not provide continuous emotional and physical support are encouraged to consider a professional doula. In addition to support in the hospital, women are encouraged to make plans for support at home in early labor, and in the days and weeks at home with the new baby.

Reshaping the Birth Environment

The environment in which birth takes place affects in profound ways how labor progresses, and how women remember their birth. In the last forty years, we have learned a great deal about both what helps and what impedes normal birth. All birth environments should provide women what they need: confidence, the freedom to find comfort in a variety of ways, and continuous emotional and physical support. To be truly supportive, the physical environment should include a place to walk; furniture such as rocking chairs, beanbags, and birth balls that promote upright positions; and access to a warm pool of water.[3] There should be one-to-one continuous nursing support as advocated by the Association of Women's Health, Obstetric and Neonatal Nurses (AWHONN).[4] Medical interventions, such as electronic fetal monitoring, intravenous fluids, and restrictions on eating, drinking, and movement which interfere with women's ability to actively work with their labors, should be used only when medically indicated.

Research continues to document the lack of benefit or harmful effect of many routine medical interventions.[5] Epidural anesthesia and induction of labor are almost routine in many hospitals, in spite of the fact that both alter the process of labor and birth in ways that are just beginning to be understood. The American College of Obstetricians and Gynecologists (ACOG) continues to recommend that induction be done only for medical indications, and that epidural anesthesia be delayed until the cervix is dilated to 4–5 cm in women pregnant with their first babies.[6] Childbirth educators may be frustrated in their efforts to help women develop and maintain confidence in their ability to give birth in many current birth environments. In early pregnancy classes, women are encouraged to choose birth settings and health care providers that provide the opportunity to find comfort in a variety of ways, and provide for continuous emotional and physical support. In Lamaze classes women learn how to minimize the possible negative effects of the birth environment and maximize the ways in which they can insure a full range of comfort and support options. Forty years ago, Lamaze education set the stage for allowing fathers in labor and delivery rooms. Lamaze is now committed to creating birth environments that provide a full range of

options for birth, including the freedom and support that
women need to have a normal birth.

Respecting the Mother/Baby Connection

Unlike forty years ago, Lamaze pays attention to the early
newborn period, viewing birth and the hours and days
immediately after birth as important influences on parenting.

The first minutes and hours after birth are critical for
mother and baby. Research supports the importance of
keeping mothers and babies together from the moment of
birth, and the importance of breastfeeding for mother and
baby.[5] Women and babies who experience normal birth are
primed and ready to greet each other and breastfeed effectively
in the first hours after birth. In Lamaze classes women are
encouraged to keep their babies close from the moment of
birth; to breastfeed their babies, respond to infant cues, and
understand the needs and capabilities of the newborn.

Reclaiming Normal Birth

Ultimately, the goal of Lamaze classes is that every woman
gives birth confidently, free to find comfort in a wide variety
of ways, and supported by family and health care professionals who trust that she has within her the ability to give birth.
By achieving our goal, Lamaze contributes to larger advocacy
efforts, which will, over time, make birth normal again.
Women in Lamaze classes are encouraged to make informed
choices about birth within the context of the limited options
that currently exist for most women. Lamaze International
believes that only when normal birth is again the standard
will women have the opportunity of making truly informed
choices about the birth of their babies.

Conclusion

Birth does not change but, over time, the environment in
which birth takes place does change, and our understanding
of both the simplicity and the complexity of birth deepens.
As a result, Lamaze preparation for birth has evolved and
will continue to evolve. The Lamaze Philosophy of Birth,
supported by an ever-growing body of research,[5] provides
direction for today's Lamaze preparation for birth. The
Lamaze Certified Childbirth Educator promotes, protects,
and supports every woman's right to give birth, confident in

her own ability, free to find comfort in a wide variety of ways, and supported by her family and all members of the health care team.

Recommended Resources

Most are available from the Lamaze Bookstore, website <www.lamaze.org> or phone 877-952-6293.

Videos

- *Birth in the squatting position.* (1979).
- *Celebrate birth!* (2000). Boulder, CO: InJoy Videos.
- *Comfort measures for childbirth.* (1995). Seattle, WA: Comfort Measures for Childbirth.
- *Gentle birth choices.* (1993). Wilsonville, OR: Global Maternal/Child Health Association.
- *Giving birth and being born.* (1995). Vienna: Austria: Karin Berghammer, Dr. Regine Ahner, and Prof. Dr. Husslein.
- *The timeless way.* (1998) Boulder, CO: InJoy Videos.
- *Tried and true - A collection of labor techniques.* (2000). Boulder, CO: InJoy Videos.

Books

- Balaskas, J. (1992). *Active birth.* Harvard and Boston, MA: The Harvard Common Press.
- Kitzinger, S. (2000). *Rediscovering birth.* New York, NY: Pocket Books.
- Enkin, M., et al. (2000). *A guide to effective care in pregnancy and childbirth.* New York, NY: Oxford University Press.
- Nichols, F. & Humenick, S. (2000). *Childbirth education: Practice, research, and theory* (second edition). Philadelphia, PA: W.B. Saunders.
- Simkin, P., & Ancheta, R. (2000). *The labor progress handbook.* Malden, MA: Blackwell Science.

References

1. Tanzer, D. (1976). *Why natural childbirth? A psychologist's report on the benefits to mothers, fathers, and babies.* New York, NY: Schocken Books.
2. Chapman, L. (1992). *Expectant fathers' roles during labor and birth.* JOGNN, 21 (2) 114-120.
3. Flamm, B., Berwick, D., & Kabcenell, A. (1998). Reducing cesarean section rates safely: lessons from a "Breakthrough Series" collaborative, *Birth*, 25 (2) 117-124.
4. AWHONN (Association of Women's Health, Obstetric, and Neonatal Nurses). (2000). *AWHONN Position Statement, Issue: Professional nursing support of laboring women.* Washington, DC: AWHONN.
5. Enkin, M., et al. (2000). *A guide to effective care in pregnancy and childbirth.* New York, NY: Oxford University Press.
6. American College of Obstetricians and Gynecologists (ACOG). (2001). *Evaluation of cesarean delivery.* Washington, DC: ACOG.

Adopted by Lamaze International Education Council Governing Body/August 2001. © Lamaze International 2001.

Visit <www.lamaze.org> to learn more about Lamaze International and to locate a Lamaze certified childbirth educator in your area.

Breastfeeding Is Priceless: No Substitute for Human Milk

Human milk is unique. Superior nutrients and beneficial substances found in human milk cannot be duplicated. Breastfeeding provides optimum health; nutritional, immuno-logical, and developmental benefits to children; and protection from postpartum complications and future disease for mothers.

Introduction

The World Health Organization, health care associations, and government health agencies affirm the scientific evidence of the clear superiority of human milk and of the hazards of artificial milk products. The World Health Organization recommends that mothers exclusively breastfeed their infants for at least the first six months, continuing breastfeeding for two years and beyond.[1] Human milk provides optimal benefits for all infants, including premature and sick newborns. The American Academy of Pediatrics encourages pediatricians to promote, protect, and support breastfeeding in their individual practices as well as in hospitals, medical schools, communities, and the nation.[2]

Although more U.S. mothers are initially breastfeeding their infants, in 2001 less than half of mothers who initiated breastfeeding did so exclusively (without supplementing with artificial milk or cow's milk) and less than one in five were breastfeeding exclusively at six months.[3] A Healthy People 2010 goal is to have three-quarters of mothers initiate breastfeeding at birth, half of them breastfeed until at least the fifth or sixth month, and one-fourth to breastfeed their babies through the end of the first year.[4]

Benefits of Breastfeeding for Children

Enhanced Immune System and Resistance to Infections

The infant's immune system is not fully mature until about two years of age. Human milk contains an abundance of infection fighting factors that are transferred to the child, including agents that act against viruses, bacteria, and intestinal parasites. Breastfeeding reduces the incidence of respiratory infections, ear infections, pneumonia, diarrhea, and urinary tract infections. Breastfeeding also helps protect against sudden infant death syndrome (SIDS). Human milk contains factors that enhance the immune response to polio, tetanus, diphtheria, and influenza.

Protection Against Chronic Disease

Exclusive breastfeeding for a minimum of four months decreases the risk of type 1 diabetes (insulin-dependent diabetes mellitus) for children with a family history of diabetes. Exclusive breastfeeding for a minimum of four months decreases the incidence of asthma and eczema. Anti-inflammatory factors in human milk reduce the incidence of bowel diseases such as Crohn's disease and ulcerative colitis. Breastfed children are also less likely to develop Hodgkin's disease or leukemia in childhood.

Nutritional, Physical, and Mental Benefits

Human milk is *the* ideally balanced and easily digested form of infant nutrition. Human milk is less stressful on immature infant kidneys and contains lipids and enzymes that promote efficient digestion and enhance nutrient absorption. The composition of human milk changes over the course of a feed, the day, and over time to accommodate the changing needs of the growing child. Breastfeeding reduces the risk of childhood obesity. Breastfed children gain less weight and are leaner at one year than formula-fed children. Human milk contains long-chain polyunsaturated fatty acids important for brain growth. School age children who were breastfed score higher on cognitive and IQ tests and tests of visual acuity. Breastfeeding also decreases the incidence of dental cavities and the need for orthodontistry.

Benefits of Breastfeeding for Premature Infants
Mothers of premature infants produce milk that is higher in protein and other nutrients than milk produced by mothers of full-term infants. Human milk contains an enzyme that helps the baby digest fat more efficiently. Breastfeeding premature infants helps to protect them against gastrointestinal and infectious disease. Human milk enhances brain stem maturation in premature infants and raises childhood IQ test scores. Breastfeeding the premature infant also reduces hospital costs and length of hospital stay.

Benefits of Breastfeeding for the Mother
Women who start breastfeeding immediately benefit from an increased level of oxytocin, a hormone that stimulates uterine contractions lowering the risk for postpartum bleeding. Women who breastfeed are more likely to lose their pregnancy weight and less likely to become obese. Breastfeeding reduces the risk of ovarian and pre-menopausal breast cancer, heart disease, and osteoporosis. The more months women breastfeed over their lifetime, the greater the protection. Exclusive breastfeeding delays the return of the menstrual cycle for twenty to thirty weeks and may lower the risk of anemia.

The Cost of Not Breastfeeding
U.S. families spend 2 billion dollars a year on human milk substitutes such as artificial milk otherwise known as formula. It costs an additional 1.3 billion dollars to cover sick-child office visits and prescriptions for respiratory infections, ear infections, and diarrhea in non-breastfed infants during the first year. In the first year of life, it will cost more than 25 thousand dollars to treat lower-respiratory infections in one thousand never-breastfed infants compared with one thousand infants exclusively breastfed for at least three months. The excess cost of treating type 1 diabetes (insulin-dependent diabetes mellitus) in formula-fed children is more than 1 trillion dollars. Private and government insurers spend

a minimum of 3.6 billion dollars a year to treat medical conditions and diseases preventable by breastfeeding.

Formula has a long history of recalls for bacterial contamination or mis-manufacture that have in many cases resulted in instances of illness, permanent injury, or death. Information on formula recalls is available at: http://www.salerts.com/rcls/category/child.htm.

References

1. U.S. Department of Health and Human Services. HHS Blueprint for Action on Breastfeeding, Washington, D.C. Office of Women's Health, 2000. http://www.cdc.gov/breastfeeding/report-blueprint.htm
2. American Academy of Pediatrics Policy Statement, Work Group on Breastfeeding. Breastfeeding and the Use of Human Milk (RE9729). Pediatrics 1997; 1035-1039. http://www.aap.org/policy/re9729.html
3. Ryan, A. S. Breastfeeding continues to increase into the new millennium. Pediatrics 2002; 110: 1103-1109.
4. U.S. Department of Health and Human Services. Healthy People 2010, Washington, D.C. Office of Disease Prevention and Health Promotion, 2002. http://www.healthypeople.gov

Other Sources

1. United States Breastfeeding Committee. Benefits of breastfeeding Raleigh, NC: United States Breastfeeding Committee; 2002. www.breastfeeding.org
2. United States Breastfeeding Committee. Economic benefits of breastfeeding. Raleigh, NC: United States Breastfeeding Committee; 2002. www.breastfeeding.org
3. Walker, Marsha, ed. Selling Out Mothers and Babies: Marketing of Breastmilk Substitutes in the USA. Weston, MA: National Alliance for Breastfeeding Advocacy, 2001.

The information provided in this position paper has been adopted from The Coalition for Improving Maternity Services (CIMS). The Coalition for Improving Maternity Services, a United Nations recognized NGO, is a collaborative effort of numerous individuals, leading researchers, and more than fifty organizations representing over ninety thousand members. Promoting a wellness model of maternity care that will improve birth outcomes and substantially reduce costs, CIMS developed the Mother-Friendly Childbirth Initiative in 1996. A consensus document that has been recognized as an important model for improving the healthcare and well being of children beginning at birth, the Mother-Friendly Childbirth Initiative has been translated into several languages and is gaining support around the world.

THE HAZARDS OF CESAREAN SURGERY FOR THE MOTHER AND BABY

Introduction

Lamaze International is concerned about the dramatic increase and ongoing overuse of cesarean section. Every year since 1983 no fewer than one in five American women has given birth via major abdominal surgery[7,15,33] Today more than one in four or 25 percent of women have a cesarean for the birth of their baby.[15] The rate for first-time mothers may approach one in three.[9] Studies show that the cesarean rate could safely be halved.[11] The World Health Organization recommends no more than a 10 to 15 percent cesarean rate.[35] With a million women having cesarean surgery every year, this means that if the cesarean rate were halved, five hundred thousand fewer women annually would have this operation.

No evidence supports the idea that cesareans are as safe as vaginal birth for mother or baby. In fact, the increase in cesarean deliveries risks the health and well being of child-bearing women and their babies.

For elective repeat cesarean, the consensus of dozens of studies totaling tens of thousands of women is that elective repeat cesarean section is riskier for the mother and not any safer for the baby.[25,28,29] Recent studies used to conclude otherwise are both seriously flawed and have been misrepresented in the media.[12]

In addition to the hazards of cesarean section per se, the risks of certain complications increase with accumulating surgeries. Studies also show that with a history of previous cesarean, seven out of ten women or more who are allowed to labor without undue restrictions will give birth vaginally, thus ending their exposure to the dangers of cesarean section.[13]

Hazards of Cesarean Section to the Mother

Women run four to seven times the risk of death from the cesarean surgery itself compared with vaginal birth.[14,16,30] Complications during and after the surgery include surgical injury to the bladder, uterus and blood vessels (2 per 100),[31] hemorrhage (1 to 6 women per 100 require a blood transfusion),[31] anesthesia accidents, blood clots in the legs (6 to 20 per 1000),[31] pulmonary embolism (1 to 2 per 1000),[31] paralyzed bowel (10 to 20 per 100 mild cases, 1 in 100 severe),[31] and infection (up to 50 times more common).[1] One in ten women report difficulties with normal activities two months after the birth,[24] and one in four report pain at the incision site as a major problem.[9] One in fourteen still report incisional pain six months or more after delivery.[9] Twice as many women require rehospitalization as women having normal vaginal birth.[20]

Especially with unplanned cesarean surgery, women are more likely to experience negative emotions, including lower self-esteem, a sense of failure, loss of control, and disappointment. They may develop postpartum depression or post-traumatic stress syndrome.[9,22,26,32] Some mothers express dominant feelings of fear and anxiety about their cesarean as long as five years later.[18] Women having cesarean sections are less likely to decide to become pregnant again.[18]

As is true of all abdominal surgery, internal scar tissue can cause pelvic pain, pain during sexual intercourse, and bowel problems. Reproductive consequences compared with vaginal birth include increased infertility,[18] miscarriage,[17] placenta previa (placenta overlies the cervix),[21] placental abruption (the placenta detaches partially or completely before the birth),[21] and premature birth.[8] Even in women planning repeat cesarean, uterine rupture occurs at a rate of 1 in 500 versus 1 in 10,000 in women with no uterine scar.[28]

Hazards of Cesarean Section to the Baby

Especially with planned cesarean, some babies will inadvertently be delivered prematurely.[1] Babies born even slightly before they are ready may experience breathing and breast-feeding problems.[23] One to two babies per 100 will be cut during the surgery.[34] Studies comparing elective cesarean section or cesarean section for reasons unrelated to the baby with vaginal birth find that babies are 50 percent more likely to have low Apgar scores, five times more likely to require assistance with breathing, and five times more likely to be admitted to intermediate or intensive care.[4] Babies born after elective cesarean section are more than four times as likely to develop persistent pulmonary hypertension compared with babies born vaginally.[19] Persistent pulmonary hypertension is life threatening.

Mothers are more likely to have difficulties forming an attachment with the infant.[22,26] This may be because women are less likely to hold and breastfeed their infants after birth and have rooming-in and because of the difficulties of caring for an infant while recovering from major surgery. Babies are less likely to be breastfed.[9] The adverse health consequences of formula feeding are numerous and can be severe.

Hazards of Elective Repeat Cesarean Section
Elective cesarean section carries twice the risk of maternal death compared with vaginal birth.[10] Old scar tissue increases the likelihood of surgical injury. One more woman in every 100 with a history of more than one cesarean will have an ectopic pregnancy (embryo implants outside the womb).[17] Hemorrhage associated with ectopic pregnancy is one of the leading causes of maternal death in the U.S.[6]

Compared with women with no uterine scar, women have more than four times the risk of placenta previa with one prior cesarean, seven times the risk with two to three prior cesareans, and forty-five times the risk with four or more prior cesareans.[3] Placenta previa more than doubles the chance of the baby dying and increases the rate of preterm birth more than six-fold.[8]

Compared with women with prior births and no previous cesareans, women with one prior cesarean or more have as much as three times the risk of placental abruption.[17] With placental abruption, 6 in every 100 babies will die, and 3 in 10 will be born too early.[21] The odds of placenta accreta (placenta grows into or even through the uterus) jump from 1 in 1,000 with one prior cesarean to 1 in 100 with more than one prior cesarean.[5] Nearly all women with this complication will require a hysterectomy, nearly half will have a massive hemorrhage, and as many as 1 in 11 babies and 1 in 14 mothers will die.[27] The incidence of placenta accreta has increased ten-fold in the last fifty years and now occurs in 1 in 2,500 births.[2]

Women having elective repeat cesareans are more likely to experience hemorrhage requiring transfusion, blood clots, and infection.[25,28,29] Postpartum recovery after repeat cesarean section is even more difficult when there is another child or children to care for.

References

ACOG. Evaluation of Cesarean Delivery. Washington, DC: ACOG, 2000.

ACOG. Placenta accreta. Committee Opinion No. 266, Jan 2002.

Ananth CV, Smulian JC, and Vintzileos AM. The association of placenta previa with history of cesarean delivery and abortion: a metaanalysis. Am J Obstet Gynecol 1997;177(5):1071-8.

Annibale DJ et al. Comparative neonatal morbidity of abdominal and vaginal deliveries after uncomplicated pregnancies. Arch Pediatr Adolesc Med 1995;149(8):862-7.

Asakura H and Myers SA. More than one previous cesarean delivery: a 5-year experience with 435 patients. Obstet Gynecol 1995;85(6):924-9.

Centers for Disease Control. Achievements in public health, 1900-1999: healthier mothers and babies. MMWR 1999: 48(38);849-58.

Centers for Disease Control. National Hospital Discharge Survey of the National Center for Health Statistics, Table 1, 1990.

Crane JM, van den Hof MC, Dodds L, Armson BA, Liston R. Neonatal outcomes with placenta previa. Obstet Gynecol 1999; 93(4):541-4.

Declercq ER, Sakala C, Corry MP. Listening to Mothers: Report of the First National U.S. Survey of Women's Childbearing Experiences. New York: Maternity Center Association, Oct 2002.

Enkin M et al. A Guide to Effective Care in Pregnancy and Childbirth. 3d ed. Oxford: Oxford University Press, 2000.

Goer H. Cesareans: Everything you need to know. http://www.parentsplace.com/expert/birthguru/articles/0,10335,243386_241096,00.html

Goer H. "Spin-doctoring" the research. Birth 2003;30(2):124-9.

Goer H. The Thinking Woman's Guide to a Better Birth. New York: Perigee Books, 1999, p 169. Hall MH. Commentary: confidential enquiry into maternal death. Br J Obstet Gynaecol 1990;97:752-3.

Hamilton BE, Martin JA, and Sutton PD al. Births: preliminary data for 2002. Nat Vital Stat Rep 2002;51(11). Harper MA et al. Pregnancy-related death and health care services. Obstet Gynecol 2003;102(2):273-8.

Hemminki E and Merilainen J. Long-term effects of cesarean sections: ectopic pregnancies and placental problems. Am J Obstet Gynecol 1996;174(5):1569-74.

Jolly J, Walker J, and Bhabra K. Subsequent obstetric performance related to primary mode of delivery. Br J Obstet Gynaecol 1999;106(3):227-32.

Levine EM et al. Mode of delivery and risk of respiratory diseases in newborns.Obstet Gynecol 2001;97(3):439-42.

Lydon-Rochelle M et al. Association between method of delivery and maternal rehospital-ization. JAMA 2000;283:2411-6.

Lydon-Rochelle M et al. First-birth cesarean and placental abruption or previa at second birth. Obstet Gynecol 2001;97(5 Pt 1):765-9.

Lydon-Rochelle MT, Holt VL, and Martin DP. Delivery method and self-reported postpartum general health status among primiparous women. Paediatric Perinatal Epidemiology 2001;15:232-40.

March of Dimes. Medical references: preterm birth. http://www.marchofdimes.com/printableArticles/681_1157.asp?printable=true

Miovich SM et al. Major concerns of women after cesarean delivery. J Obstet Gynecol Neonatal Nurs 1994;23(1):53-9.

Mozurkewich EL and Hutton EK. Elective repeat cesarean delivery versus trial of labor: a meta-analysis of the literature from 1989 to 1999. Am J Obstet Gynecol 2000:183:1187-97.

Mutryn C. Psychosocial impact of cesarean section on the family: a literature review. Soc Sci Med 1993;37(10):1271-81.

O'Brien JM, Barton JR, and Donaldson ES. The management of placenta percreta: conservative and operative strategies. Am J Obstet Gynecol 1996;175(6):1632-8.

Rageth JC, Juzi C, and Grossenbacher H. Delivery after previous cesarean: a risk evaluation. Swiss Working Group of Obstetric and Gynecologic Institutions. Obstet Gynecol 1999;93(3):332-7.

Roberts RG, Bell HS, Wall EM, et al. Trial of labor or repeated cesarean section: The woman's choice. Arch Fam Med 1997;6:120-125.

Schuitemaker N et al. Maternal mortality after cesarean in The Netherlands. Acta Obstet Gynecol Scand 1997;76(4):332-4.

Shearer EL. Cesaran section: medical benefits and costs. Soc Sci Med 1993;37(10):1223-31.

Soet JE, Brack GA, and Dilorio C. Prevalence and predictors of women's experience of psychological trauma during childbirth. Birth 2003;30(1):36-46.

U.S. Department of Health and Human Services. Rates of cesarean delivery—United States, 1991. MMWR 1993;42(15):285-300.

van Ham MA, van Dongen PW, Mulder J. Maternal consequences of caesarean section. A retrospective study of intra-operative and postoperative maternal complications of cesarean section during a 10-year period. Eur J Obstet Gynecol Reprod Biol 1997;74(1):1-6.

World Health Organization. Appropriate technology for birth. Lancet 1985;2(8452):436-437.

The information provided in this position paper has been adopted from The Coalition for Improving Maternity Services (CIMS). The Coalition for Improving Maternity Services, a United Nations recognized NGO, is a collaborative effort of numerous individuals, leading researchers, and more than fifty organizations representing over ninety thousand members. Promoting a wellness model of maternity care that will improve birth outcomes and substantially reduce costs, CIMS developed the Mother-Friendly Childbirth Initiative in 1996. A consensus document that has been recognized as an important model for improving the healthcare and well being of children beginning at birth, the Mother-Friendly Childbirth Initiative has been translated into several languages and is gaining support around the world.

Appendix E
THE DOULA'S CONTRIBUTION
TO MODERN MATERNITY CARE

The birth of each baby has a long lasting impact on the physical and mental health of mother, baby and family. In the twentieth century, we have witnessed vast improvements in the safety of childbirth, and now efforts to improve psychosocial outcomes are receiving greater attention.

The importance of fostering relationships between parents and infants cannot be overemphasized, since these early relationships largely determine the future of each family, and also of society as a whole. The quality of emotional care received by the mother during labor, birth, and immediately afterwards is one vital factor that can strengthen or weaken the emotional ties between mother and child.[1-5] Furthermore, when women receive continuous emotional support and physical comfort throughout childbirth, their obstetric outcomes may improve.[6-11]

Women have complex needs during childbirth. In addition to the safety of modern obstetrical care, and the love and companionship provided by their partners, women need consistent, continuous reassurance, comfort, encouragement and respect. They need individualized care based on their circumstances and preferences. The role of the doula encompasses the non-clinical aspects of care during childbirth.

This paper presents the position of DONA on the desirability of the presence of a doula at childbirth, with references to the medical and social sciences literature. It also explains the role of the doula in relation to the woman's partner, the nurse, and medical care providers. This paper does not discuss the postpartum doula, who provides practical help, advice, and support to families in the weeks following childbirth.

Role of the Doula

In nearly every culture throughout history, women have been surrounded and cared for by other women during childbirth.[12] Artistic representations of birth throughout the world usually include at least two other women, surrounding and supporting the birthing woman. One of these women is the midwife, who is responsible for the safe passage of the mother and baby; the other woman or women are behind or beside the mother, holding and comforting her. The modern doula is a manifestation of the woman beside the mother.

Doulas are trained and experienced in childbirth, although they may or may not have given birth themselves. The doula's role is to provide physical, emotional, and informational support to women and their partners during labor and birth. The doula offers help and advice on comfort measures such as breathing, relaxation, movement and positioning. She also assists families to gather information about the course of their labor and their options. Perhaps the most crucial role of the doula is providing continuous emotional reassurance and comfort.

Doulas specialize in non-medical skills and do not perform clinical tasks, such as vaginal exams or fetal heart rate monitoring. Doulas do not diagnose medical conditions, offer second opinions, or give medical advice. Most importantly, doulas do not make

---

Labor Support Terminology

The terminology describing labor support can be confusing. When a person uses any of the terms below to describe herself, she may need to clarify what she means by the term.

- *doula*: a Greek word meaning "woman's servant." In labor support terminology, *doula* refers to a supportive companion (not a friend or loved one) professionally trained to provide labor support. She performs no clinical tasks. *Doula* also refers to lay women who are trained or experienced in providing postpartum care (mother and newborn care, breastfeeding support and advice, cooking, child care, errands, and light cleaning) for the new family. To distinguish between the two types of doulas, one may refer to *birth doulas* and *postpartum doulas*.
- *monitrice*: a French word originally used by Fernand Lamaze to refer to a specially trained nurse or midwife who provides nursing care and assessment, in addition to labor support. Today, *monitrice* is often used as a synonym for *birth assistant* or *labor assistant*.
- *labor support professional, labor support specialist, labor companion*: synonyms of *birth doula*.
- *birth assistant, labor assistant*: sometimes these terms are used as synonyms for *doula*, but also may refer to lay women who are trained to assist a midwife (vaginal exams, set up for the birth, fetal heart checks, etc.) as well as to provide some labor support.

decisions for their clients; they do not project their own values and goals onto the laboring woman.[13]

The doula's goal is to help the woman have a safe and satisfying childbirth as the woman defines it. When a doula is present, some women feel less need for pain medications, or may postpone them until later in labor; however, many women choose or need pharmacological pain relief. It is not the role of the doula to discourage the mother from her choices. The doula helps her become informed about various options, including the risks, benefits and accompanying precautions or interventions for safety. Doulas can help maximize the benefits of pain medications while minimizing their undesirable side effects. The comfort and reassurance offered by the doula are beneficial regardless of the use of pain medications.

The Doula and the Partner Work Together

The woman's partner (the baby's father or another loved one) plays an essential role in providing support for the woman. A doula cannot make some of the unique contributions that the partner makes, such as intimate knowledge of the woman and love for her and her child. The doula is there in addition to, not instead of, the partner. Ideally, the doula and the partner make the perfect support team for the woman, complementing each other's strengths.

In the 1960's, the earliest days of fathers' involvement in childbirth, the expectation was that they would be intimately involved as advisors, coaches and decision-makers for the woman. This turned out to be an unrealistic expectation for most men because they had little prior knowledge of birth or medical procedures and little confidence or desire to ask questions of medical staff. In addition, some men felt helpless and distressed over the women's pain and were not able to provide the constant reassurance and nurturing that women need. With a doula present, the pressure on the father is decreased and he can participate at his own comfort level. Fathers often feel relieved when they can rely on a doula for help; they enjoy the experience more. For those fathers who want to play an active support role, the doula assists and guides them in effective ways to help their loved ones in labor. Partners other than fathers (lovers, friends, family members) also appreciate the doula's support, reassurance and assistance.

Doulas as Members of the Maternity Care Team

Each person involved in the care of the laboring woman contributes to her emotional well-being. However, doctors, nurses, and midwives are primarily responsible for the health and well-being of the mother and baby. Medical care providers must assess the condition of the mother and fetus, diagnose and treat complications as they arise, and focus on a safe delivery of the baby. These priorities rightly take precedence over the non-medical psychosocial needs of laboring women.

The doula helps ensure that these needs are met while enhancing communication and understanding between the woman or couple and the staff. Many doctors, midwives and nurses appreciate the extra attention given to their patients and the greater satisfaction expressed by women who were assisted by a doula.[14]

Questions to Ask a Doula

To discover the specific training, experience and services offered by anyone who provides labor support, potential clients, nursing supervisors, physicians, midwives, and others should ask the following questions of that person.

- What training have you had? (If a doula is certified, you might consider checking with the organization.)
- Tell me about your experience with birth, personally and as a doula.
- What is your philosophy about childbirth and supporting women and their partners through labor?
- May we meet to discuss our birth plans and the role you will play in supporting me through childbirth?
- May we call you with questions or concerns before and after the birth?
- When do you try to join women in labor? Do you come to our home or meet us at the hospital?
- Do you meet with us after the birth to review the labor and answer questions?
- Do you work with one or more back up doulas for times when you are not available? May we meet them?
- What are your fee and refund policies?

Research Findings

In the late 1970's, when Drs. John Kennell and Marshall Klaus investigated ways to enhance maternal-infant bonding they found, almost accidentally, that introducing a doula into the labor room not only improved the bond between mother and infant, but also seemed to decrease the incidence of complications.[6,7] Since their original studies, published in 1980 and 1986, numerous scientific trials have been conducted in many countries, comparing usual care with usual care plus a doula. Table 1 summarizes the findings of these studies, confirming the value of the doula.

As can be seen in Table 1, obstetric outcomes were most improved and intervention rates most dramatically lowered by doulas in settings where the women had no loved ones present, the intervention rates were routinely high (as indicated by the data for the control groups), and the doulas were not health care professionals.

Table 1. Summary of findings of randomized controlled trials of doulas or health care professionals acting as doulas.
Key to abbreviations: n/a = not assessed; c/s = cesarean section rate; mod = moderate; NICU = neonatal intensive care unit admission; PPD = postpartum depression; + = positive; E = experimental (supported); C = control group; O = observed group

Author, date of study	Loved ones present?	Epi-dural	Oxy-tocin	Forceps, V/E	C/S	Apgar <7@5 min.	NICU/inc. Newborn hosp. stay	B/F @ 4-6 wks.	mod to high PPD scores @ 6 wks	+ birth experience	+ self-image
Studies of doulas											
Sosa '80[6] E 32	N	n/a	6%*	1%	19%*	n/a	n/a	n/a	n/a	n/a	n/a
C 95	N	n/a	17%	4%	27%	n/a	n/a	n/a	n/a	n/a	n/a
Klaus '86[7] E 186	N	n/a	2%*	1%	7%*	2%	2%	n/a	n/a	n/a	n/a
C 279	N	n/a	13%	3%	17%	3%	7%	n/a	n/a	n/a	n/a
Hofmeyr '91[1] & Wolman '93[2] E 92	N	n/a	8%	n/a	12%	n/a	n/a	51%*	11%*	58.7%	59%*
C 97	N	n/a	10%	n/a	14.4%	n/a	n/a	29%	59%	24%	24%
Studies of trained doulas											
Kennell '91[8]** E 212	N	7.8%*	17%*	8.2%*	8/5*	n/a	10.4%*	n/a	n/a	n/a	n/a
O 200	N	22.6%	23%	21.3%	13%	n/a	17%	n/a	n/a	n/a	n/a
C 204	N	55.3%	43.6%	26.3%	18%	n/a	24%	n/a	n/a	n/a	n/a
Kennell '93[9] & '94[10] E 300	Y	67%	n/a	n/a	15%*	n/a	15.4%*	n/a	n/a	n/a	n/a
C 270	Y	76%	n/a	n/a	24.8%	n/a	24.4%	n/a	n/a	n/a	n/a
Gordon '98[17] E 169	Y	52.7%	61.5%	18.3%	16.6%	n/a	n/a	87.9%	n/a	43.5%*	54.6%*
C 209	Y	62.5%	59.8%	27.2%	15.3%	n/a	n/a	84.2%	n/a	31.7%	44.4%
Studies of nurses, midwives, or students acting as doulas											
Langer '98[3] E 361	N	83%	n/a	2.8%	24%	2.8%	n/a	12%*	n/a	37.6%	39%
C 363	N	87%	n/a	3.4%	27%	4.5%	n/a	7%	n/a	28.8%	38%
Hodnett '89[18], '89[19] E 72	Y	61%*	43%	18%	17%	n/a	n/a	n/a	n/a	n/a	n/a
C 73	Y	80%	22%	24%	18%	n/a	n/a	n/a	n/a	n/a	n/a
Cogan '88[20] E 20	Y	30%	43%	n/a	10%	0%	43%	n/a	n/a	n/a	n/a
C 14	Y	66%	64%	n/a	14%	36%	57%	n/a	n/a	n/a	n/a

* statistically significant difference
** This study consisted of three groups, the first two of which were randomly allocated: doula-accompanied woman (E); observed women (O) (a silent observer was in the room behind a curtain); and control (C), who received usual care without a doula or an observer. Group C was added after the trial, when it became clear that the presence of a silent observer improved outcomes, possibly by influencing staff behavior or by ensuring that the women were not alone.

Services and Costs

There are two basic types of doula services: independent doula practices and hospital/agency doula programs. Independent doulas are employed directly by the parents. They usually have telephone contact and at least one prenatal meeting with their clients to establish a relationship. When labor begins, the doula arrives and stays with the woman until after the birth. A postpartum meeting to process the birth is usually included in the doula's service. Most doulas charge a flat fee for their services, and many base their fees on a sliding scale.

Some doula programs are associated with or administered by a hospital or community service agency. The doulas may be volunteers or paid employees of the hospital or agency. These programs vary widely in their design. In some, the hospital or agency contracts with an independent community-based doula group to provide the doulas. Others train and employ their own staff of doulas. Payment of the doula may come from the institution, the client, or it may be shared by the two. Some hospital/agency services are set up as on call doula services. A rotating call schedule ensures that there are one or more doulas available at all times. They meet the client for the first time and establish their relationship during labor.

Other hospital/agency doula programs make doula services available to expectant mothers or couples, who may meet and choose their doula, or have one assigned to them, along with a backup doula. They may work with their doula in much the same way that private doulas and clients work together.

There is growing third party reimbursement for labor support. Grant funding is often available, and some Medicaid-funded health agencies have contracts with doula organizations to support women in poverty and women with special needs. At present, however, most doula care is paid for directly by the client.

Training and Certification of Doulas

Doula training focuses on the emotional needs of women in labor, and non-medical physical and emotional comfort measures. Generally, training programs require some prior knowledge of childbirth, and consist of an intensive two or three day seminar, including hands-on practice of such skills as relaxation, breathing, positioning and movements to reduce pain and enhance labor progress, massage, and other comfort measures.

Certification is offered by several local, national, and international organizations. For certification, most programs require a background of work and education in the maternity field, or observation of a series of childbirth classes; a doula training course; background reading; and a written exam or essay that demonstrates understanding of the integral concepts of labor support. Positive evaluations from clients, doctors or midwives and nurses are also required.

Summary and Conclusion

In summary, the doula is emerging as a positive contribution to the care of women in labor. By attending to the women's emotional needs, some obstetric outcomes are improved. Just as importantly, early mother-infant relationships and breast-feeding are enhanced. Women's satisfaction with their birth experiences and even their self-esteem appears to improve when a doula has assisted them through childbirth.

Analysis of the numerous scientific trials of labor support led the prestigious scientific group, The Cochrane Collaboration's Pregnancy and Childbirth Group in Oxford, England to state: "Given the clear benefits and no known risks associated with intrapartum support, every effort should be made to ensure that all labouring women receive support, not only from those close to them but also from specially trained caregivers. This support should include continuous presence, the provision of hands-on comfort, and encouragement."[15]

References

1. Hofmeyr J, Nikodem VC, Wolman WL, Chalmers BE, Kramer T. "Companionship to modify the clinical birth environment: effects on progress and perceptions of labour, and breastfeeding," Br J Obstet Gynaecol, 98:756-764, 1991.
2. Wolman WL, Chalmers B, Hofmeyr J. Nikodem VC. "Postpartum depression and companionship in the clinical birth environment: a randomized, controlled study," Am J Obstet Gynecol, 168:1388-1393, 1993.
3. Langer A, Campero L, Garcia C, Reynoso S. "Effects of Psychosocial support during labour and childbirth on breast feeding, medical interventions, and mothers' well-being in a Mexican public hospital: a randomised clinical trial." Br J Obstet Gynaecol, 105:1056-1063, 1998.

4. Martin S, Landry S, Steelman L, Kennell JH, McGrath S. "The effect of doula support during labor on mother-infant interaction at 2 months," Infant Behav Devel, 21:556, 1998.
5. Landry SH, McGrath SK, Kennell JH, Martin S, Steelman L, "The effects of doula support during labor on mother-infant interaction at 2 months," Pediatric Res, 43(4):Part 11, 13 A, 1998.
6. Sosa R, Kennell JH, Klaus MH, Robertson S, Urrutia J. "The effect of a supportive companion on perinatal problems, length of labor, and mother-infant interaction," N Engl J Med, 303:597-600, 1980.
7. Klaus MH, Kennell JH, Robertson SS, Sosa R. "Effects of social support during parturition on maternal and infant morbidity," Br Med J, 293:585-587, 1986.
8. Kennell JH, Klaus MH, McGrath SK, Robertson S, Hinkley C. "Continuous emotional support during labor in a US hospital: a randomized controlled trial," JAMA, 265:2197-2201, 1991.
9. Kennell JH, McGrath SK "Labor support by a doula for middle-income couples; the effect on cesarean rates," Pediatric Res, 32:12A, 1993.
10. Kennell J H. "The effects of continuous emotional support for couples during labor," Presentation at the first international conference of Doulas of North America, Seattle, WA, July 22, 1994.
11. McGrath SK, Kennell JH, "Induction of labor and doula support," Pediatric Res, 43(4):Part II, 14A, 1998.
12. Ashford JI. George Engelmann and Primitive Birth. Janet Isaacs Ashford, Solana Beach, CA, 1988.
13. Doulas of North America, Code of Ethics and Standards of Practice, DONA, Seattle, WA, 1992.
14. Gilliland AL. "Commentary: nurses, doulas, and childbirth educators," J Perinatal Ed, 7:18-24, 1998.
15. Hodneft ED. "Support from caregivers during childbirth." (Cochrane Review) In the Cochrane Library, Issue 2. Oxford Update Software, 1998. Updated quarterly.
16. Hommel F. "Natural childbirth: nurses in private practice as monitrices," Amer J of Nursing, 69:1446-50, 1969.
17. Gordon NP, Walton D, McAdam E, Derman J, Gallitero G, Garrett L. "Effects of providing hospital-based doulas in health maintenance organization hospitals." Obstet Gynecol, 93(3):422-426, 1999.
18. Hodnett ED, Osborn RW. "A randomised trial of the effects of monitrice support during labor: mothers' views two to four weeks postpartum," Birth, 16:177-183,1989.
19. Hodnett ED, Osborn RW. "Effects of continuous intrapartum professional support on childbirth outcomes," Res Nurs Hlth, 12:289-297,1989.
20. Cogan R, Spinnato JA. "Social support during premature labor: effects on labor and the newborn," J Psychosom Obstet Gynaecol, 8:209-216,1988.

This paper was written by Penny Simkin and Kelli Way, and reviewed and edited by Connie Livingston, Director of Publications, and the 1998 DONA Board of Directors.

For more information about doulas, contact:
Doulas of North America (DONA)
888-788-DONA
www.DONA.org

To purchase copies of this paper, contact DONA at the number above or order them on-line in the Doula Boutique on the DONA website at www.dona.org.

REFERENCES

Chapter 1

1. World Health Organization Department of Reproductive Health and Research. (1999) "Care in Normal Birth: A Practical Guide." Geneva: World Health Organization, 3.
2. Declercq, E., et al. (2002) *Listening to Mothers: Report of the First National U.S. Survey of Women's Childbearing Experiences.* New York: Maternity Center Association.
3. National Center for Health Statistics, Centers for Disease Control and Prevention, Hyattsville, Md 20782; 301-458-4000, http://www.cdc.gov/nchs.
4. Enkin, M., et al. (2000) *A Guide to Effective Care in Pregnancy and Childbirth.* New York: Oxford University Press.
5. National Vital Statistics (2004).
6. See note 1 above.
7. Maternity Center Association. (2004) *What Every Pregnant Woman Needs to Know About Cesarean Section.* New York: Maternity Center Association. (Full text available at www.maternitywise.org.)
8. Kroger, M. (2004) *Impact of Birthing Practices on Breastfeeding: Protecting the Mother and Baby Continuum.* Sudbury, Ma: Jones and Bartlett Publishers.
9. Ad Council and U.S. Department of Health and Human Services. (2004) Breastfeeding Awareness Ad Campaign, www.adcouncil.org.
10. American Academy of Pediatrics. (2005) "Breastfeeding and the use of human milk." *Pediatrics.* 115, no. 2: 496–506.
11. See note 2 above.
12. Simkin, P. (1992) "Just another day in a woman's life? Nature and consistency of women's long term memories of their first birth experience." *Birth* 19:64–81.
13. Hodnett, E. (2002) "Pain and women's satisfaction with the experience of birth: A systematic review." *American Journal of Obstetrics and Gynecology* 186, no. 5:s160.
14. Knapp, L. (1996) "Childbirth satisfaction: the effect of internality and perceived control." *Journal of Perinatal Education* 5:7–15.
15. Simkin, P., interview by Jillian Hanson. "Mother-Friendly Trends." *Pregnancy Today: The Journal for Parents-To-Be.*

Chapter 2

1. Rooks, J. (1997) *Midwifery and Childbirth in America.* Philadelphia: Temple University Press, chapter 2.
2. Ibid., chapter 1.
3. Ibid., 29–32.

4. White House Conference on Child Health and Protection (1932).
5. See note 1 above.
6. Sullivan, N. (March 6, 2002) midwifeinfo.com.
7. Gaskin, I. M. (2003) *Ina May's Guide to Childbirth.* New York: Bantam, 131
8. Enkin, M., et al. (2000) *A Guide to Effective Care in Pregnancy and Childbirth.* New York: Oxford University Press.
9. Bing, E. (1996) "Lamaze Childbirth: Then and Now." *Lamaze Parents' Magazine.*
10. Jordan, B. (1975) *American Journal of Obstetrics and Gynecology* 80, no. 2:284–90.
11. Odent, M. (1984) *Birth Reborn.* New York: Pantheon Books, 50.
12. Rooks, J. (1997) *Midwifery and Childbirth in America.* Philadelphia: Temple University Press, 246–47.
13. House of Commons Health Committee. (1992) *Second Report, Maternity Services* 1. London: HMSO, xciv.
14. See www.cia.gov/cia/publications/factbook for a rank ordering of world's nations on infant mortality rates.
15. *The Cochrane Library.* Oxford: Update Software. (www.cochrane.org)
16. See note 8 above.
17. Ibid., chapter 30.
18. Ryan, K. J. (1988) "Giving Birth in America." *Family Planning Perspectives* 20:298–301.
19. See note 14 above.
20. Rooks, J. (1997) *Midwifery and Childbirth in America.* Philadelphia: Temple University Press.
21. See note 8 above.
22. Luce, B. (March 2004) "A Natural Choice." *Swarthmore.*
23. American College of Nurse-Midwives, www.midwife.org; Midwives Alliance of North America, www.mana.org.
24. See note 22 above.
25. Coalition for the Improvement of Maternity Services, www.motherfriendly.org.
26. Association of Nurse Advocates for Childbirth Solutions. Mission statement. (www.anacs.org)
27. McGhee, C. "The Value and Purpose of Labor Support." *International Doula* 11, no. 3.
28. Lamaze Institute for Normal Birth, www.normalbirth.org.
29. Birthing Project USA, 1900 T. Street, Sacramento, Ca 95814; 888-657-9790, www.birthingprojectusa.com.
30. Rogers, F. (1998) Lifetime Achievement Award acceptance speech given at the Daytime Emmy Awards ceremony.

Chapter 3

1. Flaxman, S. and P. W. Sherman. (June 2000) *The Quarterly Review of Biology* 75, no. 2:113–48.
2. England, P. and R. Horowitz. (1998) *Birthing from Within*. Albuquerque, New Mexico: Partera Press, 256.
3. Harding, R. and A. Bocking, ed. (2001) *Fetal Growth and Development*. New York: Cambridge University Press.
4. Gaskin, I. M. (2003) *Ina May's Guide to Childbirth*. New York: Bantam, 303.
5. Fernandes, O., et al. (1998) "Moderate to heavy caffeine consumption and relationship to spontaneous abortion and abnormal fetal growth: a meta-analysis." *Reproductive Toxicology* 12:435–44.
6. Enkin, M., et al. (2000) *A Guide to Effective Care in Pregnancy and Childbirth*. New York: Oxford University Press, chapter 5.

Chapter 4

1. *Rights of Childbearing Women*. New York: Maternity Center Association. (See Appendix C.)
2. World Health Organization. (1999) "Care in normal birth: Report of a technical work group." Geneva: World Health Organization.
3. Rooks, J. (1997) *Midwifery and Childbirth in America*. Philadelphia: Temple University Press, chapter 1.
4. Devitt, N. (1979) "The statistical case for the elimination of the midwife: fact versus prejudice, 1890–1935 (Parts 1 and 2)." *Women and Health* 4:(part 1) 81–96 (part 2) 169–83.
5. Enkin, M., et al. (2000) *A Guide to Effective Care in Pregnancy and Childbirth*. New York: Oxford University Press.
6. Ibid.
7. Maternity Center Association. (2003) *What Every Woman Needs to Know About Cesarean Section*. New York: Maternity Center Association.
8. Enkin, M., et al. (2000) *A Guide to Effective Care in Pregnancy and Childbirth*. New York: Oxford University Press, 251.
9. Mayberry, L., D. Clemmens, and A. De. (2002) "Epidural analgesia side effects, co-interventions, and care of women during childbirth: A systematic review." *Supplement to American Journal of Obstetrics and Gynecology*. 186, no. 5:s81–s93.
10. Enkin, M., et al. (2000) *A Guide to Effective Care in Pregnancy and Childbirth*. New York: Oxford University Press, 21.
11. Ibid.
12. Ibid.
13. Declercq, E., et al. (2002) *Listening to Mothers: Report of the First National U.S. Survey of Women's Childbearing Experiences*. New York: Maternity Center Association.

14. Rooks, J. (1997) *Midwifery and Childbirth in America*. Philadelphia: Temple University Press, 448.
15. See note 10 above.
16. Rooks, J. (1997) *Midwifery and Childbirth in America*. Philadelphia: Temple University Press, 458.
17. See note 10 above.
18. Gaskin, I. M. (2003) *Ina May's Guide to Childbirth*. New York: Bantam, 310.
19. Fein, E., CNM. Personal communication with authors.
20. Rooks, J. (1997) *Midwifery and Childbirth in America*. Philadelphia: Temple University Press, 106.
21. Rosenblatt, R. (1988) "The future of obstetrics in family practice." *Journal of Family Practice* 26:127–29.
22. Coalition for Improving Maternity Services. (2000) *Having a Baby? Ten Questions to Ask*. www.motherfriendly.org.
23. Tumblin, A. and P. Simkin. (2001) "Pregnant women's perceptions of their nurse's role during labor and birth." *Birth* 28, no. 1:52–56.
24. Hodnett, E. (2003) "Continuous support for women during childbirth." *The Cochrane Library* 3. Oxford: Update Software. (Full text available at www.maternitywise.org.)
25. Knapp, L. (1996) "Childbirth satisfaction: the effect of internality and perceived control." *Journal of Perinatal Education* 5:7–14.
26. Enkin, M., et al. (2000) *A Guide to Effective Care in Pregnancy and Childbirth*. New York: Oxford University Press, 250–51.
27. Ibid.
28. See note 13 above.
29. Enkin, M., et al. (2000) *A Guide to Effective Care in Pregnancy and Childbirth*. New York: Oxford University Press, 248–49.
30. American College of Nurse Midwives. (2003) "Criteria for Provision of Home Birth Services." *Clinical Bulletin 7*. (www.acnm.org)
31. Kitzinger, S. (2002) *Birth Your Way*. London: DK Publishers.

Chapter 5

1. Enkin, M., et al. (2000) *A Guide to Effective Care in Pregnancy and Childbirth*. New York: Oxford University Press, chapter 6.
2. Ibid.
3. Eskenazi, B. (1999) "Caffeine-filtering the facts." *New England Journal of Medicine* 341, no. 22:1688–89.
4. Raikkonen, K. (2005) "Sweet babies: Chocolate consumption during pregnancy and infant temperament at 6 months." *Early Human Development* 76:139.

5. American Academy of Pediatrics. (2005) "Policy Statement: Breastfeeding and the Use of Human Milk." *Pediatrics* 115, no. 2:496–506.
6. American Academy of Pediatrics, www.aap.org.
7. *OBGYN Headline News*. (April 15, 2004) www.obgyn.net.
8. Enkin, M., et al. (2000) *A Guide to Effective Care in Pregnancy and Childbirth*. New York: Oxford University Press, 58.
9. Wagner, M. (1994) *Pursuing the Birth Machine: The Search for Appropriate Birth Technology*. Sevenoaks, Kent, UK: ACE Graphics.
10. *USA Today*. (February 3, 2004) "Long-held prenatal beliefs challenged." 1D.
11. Enkin, M., et al. (2000) *A Guide to Effective Care in Pregnancy and Childbirth*. New York: Oxford University Press, 77.
12. Rothman, B. K., et al. (2001) *Birth by Design*. New York: Routledge, 180–98.
13. Ibid.
14. Hall, K, (September 24, 2000) "Whispers, Dreams, and Blessings: Ancient Rituals for a New Millennium." Talk given at Lamaze International Conference, Memphis, Tenn.

Chapter 7
1. Odent, M. (2003) *Birth and Breastfeeding: Discovering the needs of women during pregnancy and breastfeeding*. East Sussex, UK: Clarview Books.
2. Righard, L. and M. Alade. (1990) "Effect of delivery room routines on success of first breastfeed." *Lancet* 336, no. 8723:1105–107. (See also Delivery Self Attachment and The Amazing Talents of the Newborn in Recommended Resources.)
3. Kitzinger, S. (2000) *Rediscovering Birth*. New York: Pocket Books, 142.
4. Klaus, M., J. Kennell, and P. Klaus. (2002) *The Doula Book: How a Trained Labor Companion Can Help You Have a Shorter, Easier, and Healthier Birth*. Cambridge, Ma.: Perseus Publishing, 72.

Chapter 8
1. Kitzinger, S. (2002) *Birth Your Way*. London: Dorling Kindersley Limited, 151.
2. Kramer, M., et al. (2000) "The contribution of mild and moderate preterm birth to infant mortality." *Journal of the American Medical Association* 284, no. 7:843–49.
3. American College of Obstetricians and Gynecologists. (2000) *Planning your pregnancy and birth*. Washington, DC: ACOG.
4. American College of Obstetricians and Gynecologists. (2002) "ACOG news release: Cesarean delivery more likely with labor induction of a large baby." Washington, DC: ACOG; Sanchez-Ramos, et al. (2002) "Expectant management versus labor induction for suspected fetal macrosomia: A systematic review." *Obstetrics and Gynecology* 100, no. 5: 997–1002.
5. Alexander, J., et al. (2000) "Forty weeks and beyond: Pregnancy outcome by week of gestation." *Obstetrics and Gynecology* 96, no. 2:291–94; Enkin, M., et al. (2000) *A Guide to Effective Care in Pregnancy and Childbirth*. New York: Oxford University Press.
6. Roberts, J., et al. (1983) "The effects of maternal position on uterine contractility and efficiency." *Birth* 10:243–49.
7. Kroger, M. (2004) *Maternal positions in labor, birth, and breastfeeding. Impact of birthing practices on breastfeeding: Protecting the mother and baby continuum*. Sudbury, Ma.: Jones and Bartlett Publishers, 70.
8. Carlson, J., et al. (1986) "Maternal positions during parturition in normal labor." *Obstetrics and Gynecology* 68, no. 4:443–47.
9. Enkin, M., et al. (2000) *A Guide to Effective Care in Pregnancy and Childbirth*. New York: Oxford University Press.
10. Bloom, S., et al. (1998) "Lack of effect of walking." *The New England Journal of Medicine* 339, no. 2:117–18.
11. Declercq, E., et al. (2002) *Listening to Mothers: Report of the First National U.S. Survey of Women's Childbearing Experiences*. New York: Maternity Center Association.
12. Adachi, K., M. Shimada, and A. Usai. (2003) "The relationship between parturient's positions and perceptions of labor pain intensity." *Nursing Research* 52, no. 1:47–51.
13. Kitzinger, S. (2000) *Rediscovering Birth*. New York: Pocket Books, 99.
14. Hodnett, E. (2003) "Continuous support for women during childbirth." *The Cochrane Library* 3. Oxford: Update Software. (Full text available at www.maternitywise.org.)
15. Tumlin, A. and P. Simkin. (2001) "Pregnant women's perceptions of their nurse's role during labor and birth." *Birth* 28, no. 1:52–56.
16. Hodnett, E. (1996) "Nursing support of the laboring woman." *Journal of Obstetric, Gynecologic, and Neonatal Nursing* 25:257–64.
17. Kennell, J. Personal communication.
18. Enkin, M., et al. (2000) *A Guide to Effective Care in Pregnancy and Childbirth*. New York: Oxford University Press, chapter 50.
19. Declercq, E., et al. (2002) *Listening to Mothers: Report of the First National U.S. Survey of Women's Childbearing Experiences*. New York: Maternity Center Association.
20. O'Sullivan, G. (1994) "The stomach—fact and fantasy: eating and drinking during labour." *International Anesthesiology Clinics* 32:31–44.

21. American Society of Anesthesiologists Task Force. (1999) "Practice guidelines for preoperative fasting and the use of pharmacologic agents to reduce the risk of pulmonary aspiration: application to healthy patients undergoing elective procedures." *Anesthesiology* 90, no. 3:896–905.

22. Ibid.; American College of Obstetricians and Gynecologists. (2002) "ACOG practice bulletin: Obstetric analgesia and anesthesia." *Obstetrics and Gynecology* 100, no. 1: 177–91.

23. American College of Nurse-Midwives. (March 1999, revised February 2000) "Intrapartum Nutrition." *Clinical Bulletin* 3. http://www.midwife.org/prof/display.cfm?id=115 (accessed May 5, 2005).

24. Society of Obstetricians and Gynaecologists of Canada. (1998) *Healthy Beginnings: Guidelines for Care during Pregnancy and Childbirth.* (http://www.sogc.medical.org)

25. Enkin, M., et al. (2000) *A Guide to Effective Care in Pregnancy and Childbirth.* New York: Oxford University Press, chapter 29.

26. Begum, M., et al., ed. (1999) *Obstetrics for Postgraduates and Practitioners.* New Delhi: BI Churchill Livingstone.

27. Simkin, P. (1986a) "Stress, pain and catecholamines in labor: Part 1. A Review." *Birth* 13:227–33.

28. See note 18 above.

29. Enkin, M., et al. (2000) *A Guide to Effective Care in Pregnancy and Childbirth.* New York: Oxford University Press, chapter 30.

30. American College of Obstetricians and Gynecologists. (2005) "ACOG practice bulletin: Intrapartum fetal heart rate monitoring." *Obstetrics and Gynecology* 105, no. 5:1161–1168.

31. Association of Women's Health and Obstetric and Neonatal Nurses. (1997, 2000) "Fetal Heart Rate Monitoring Principles and Practices." Washington, DC.

32. See note 18 above.

33. Fraser, W., et al. (2003) "Amniotomy for shortening spontaneous labour." *The Cochrane Library* 2. Oxford: Update Software.

34. Enkin, M., et al. (2000) *A Guide to Effective Care in Pregnancy and Childbirth.* New York: Oxford University Press, chapter 35.

35. See note 33 above.

36. Enkin, M., et al. (2000) *A Guide to Effective Care in Pregnancy and Childbirth.* New York: Oxford University Press, 337.

37. Declercq, E., et al. (2002) *Listening to Mothers: Report of the First National U.S. Survey of Women's Childbearing Experiences.* New York: Maternity Center Association.

38. Mayberry, L., D. Clemmens, and A. De. (2002) "Epidural analgesia side effects, co-interventions, and care of women during childbirth: A systematic review." *Supplement to American*

Journal of Obstetrics and Gynecology. 186, no. 5:s81–s93.

39. Lieberman, E. and C. O'Donoghue. (2002) "Unintended effects of epidural analgesia during labor: a systematic review." *Supplement to American Journal of Obstetrics and Gynecology* 186, no. 5:s31–s68.

40. Howell, C. J. (2003) "Epidural versus non-epidural analgesia for pain relief in labor." *The Cochrane Library* 3. Oxford: Update Software.

41. Righard, L. and M. Alade. (1990) "Effect of delivery room routines on success of first breastfeed." *Lancet* 336, no. 8723:1105–107.

42. Matthiesen, A., et al. (2001) "Maternal analgesia during labor disturbs newborn behavior: Effects on breastfeeding, temperature, and crying." *Birth* 28, no. 1:5–12.

43. See note 18 above.

44. See note 37 above.

45. See note 18 above.

46. Gupta, J. and C. Nickoderm. (2000) "Maternal posture in labour." *European Journal of Obstetrics and Gynecology and Reproductive Biology* 92, no. 2:273–77; see note 18 above.

47. Johnson, N., V. Johnson, and J. Gupta. (1991) "Maternal positions during labor." *Obstetrical and Gynecological Survey* 46, no. 7:428–34.

48. See note 18 above.

49. Mayberry, L., et al. (2000) *Second-stage management: promotion of evidence-based practice and a collaborative approach to patient care.* Washington, DC: Association of Women's Health, Obstetric and Neonatal Nurses (AWHONN).

50. Anderson, G., et al. (2003) "Early skin-to-skin contact for mothers and their healthy newborn infants." *The Cochrane Library* 3. Oxford: Update Software.

51. Uvnas-Moberg, K. (1998) "Oxytocin may mediate the benefits of positive social interactions and emotions." *Psychoneuroendocrinology* 23, no. 8:819–38.

52. American Academy of Pediatrics (AAP) and American College of Obstetricians and Gynecologists (ACOG). (2002) *Guidelines for Perinatal Care.* Elk Grove, Il. and Washington, DC: AAP and ACOG; American Academy of Breastfeeding Medicine Protocol and Committee. (2003) "Clinical protocol #5: Peripartum breastfeeding management for the healthy mother and infant at term." *Academy of Breastfeeding Medicine News and Views* 9, no. 1; Association of Women's Health, Obstetric and Neonatal Nurses. (2000) *Evidence-based clinical practice guideline: Breastfeeding support: Prenatal care through the first year.* Washington, DC: AWHONN; World Health Organization (WHO). (1998) *Evidence for the 10 steps to successful breastfeeding.* Geneva, Switzerland: WHO.

53. Mikiel-Kostyra, K., J. Mazur, and I. Boltruszko. (2002) "Effect of skin-to-skin contact after delivery on duration of breastfeeding: a prospective study." *Acta Paediatrica* 91, no. 12;1301–306.

54. Christenssen, K., et al. (1992) "Temperature, metabolic adaptation and crying in healthy full-term newborns cared for skin-to-skin or in a cot." *Acta Paediatrica* 81, no. 6–7:488–93; ——— (1998) "Randomised study of skin-to-skin versus incubator care for rewarming low-risk hypothermic neonates." *Lancet* 352, no. 9134:1115; Bystrova, K., et al. (2003) "Skin-to-skin contact may reduce negative consequences of 'the stress of being born': A study on temperature in newborn infants subjected to different ward routines in St. Petersburg." *Acta Paediatrica* 92, no. 3:320–26.

55. Washington, DC: AWHONN; World Health Organization (WHO). (1998) *Evidence for the 10 steps to successful breastfeeding.* Geneva, Switzerland: WHO.

56. Christenssen, K., C. Siles, Moreno, L. Belaustequi, A., De La Fuente, et al. (1992); Christensson, K., et al. (1995). "Separation distress call in the human neonate in the absence of maternal body contact." *Acta Paediatrica* 84, no. 5:468–73; Johanson, R., et al. (1992) "Effect of post-delivery care on neonatal body temperature." *Acta Paediatrica* 81, no. 11:859–63.

57. Righard, L. and M. Alade. (1990) "Effect of delivery room routines on success of first breastfeed." *Lancet* 336, no. 8723:1105–107.

58. Gaskin, I. M. (2003) *Ina May's Guide to Childbirth.* New York: Bantam.

Chapter 9

1. Simkin, P. (2001) *The Birth Partner.* Cambridge, Ma.: Harvard Common Press.

2. Kitzinger, S. (2000) *Rediscovering Birth.* New York: Pocket Books, chapter 7.

3. Trolle, B., et al. (1991) "The effect of sterile water blocks on low back labor pain." *American Journal of Obstetrics and Gynecology* 164, no. 5:1277–281.

Chapter 10

1. Hodnett, E., et al. (2003) "Continuous support for women during childbirth." *The Cochrane Library* 3. Oxford: Update Software. (Full report available at www.maternitywise.org.)

2. Enkin, M., et al. (2000) *A Guide to Effective Care in Pregnancy and Childbirth.* New York: Oxford University Press, chapter 30.

3. Ibid., chapter 29.

4. Hawkins, J. L., et al. (1998) "Practice Guidelines for Obstetrical Anesthesia: A Report by the American Society of Anesthesiologists Task Force on Obstetrical Anesthesia."

5. Enkin, M., et al. (2000) *A Guide to Effective Care in Pregnancy and Childbirth.* New York: Oxford University Press, chapter 29.

6. Ibid., chapter 35.

7. Ibid., chapter 32.

8. Lieberman, E. and C. O'Donoghue. (2002) "Unintended effects of epidural analgesia during labor: A systematic review." *Supplement to Journal of Obstetrics and Gynecology* 186, no. 5:s31–s68.

9. Ibid.

10. Ibid.

11. See note 7 above.

12. Sakala, C., M. Corry, and H. Goer. (2004) *Vaginal Birth and Cesarean Birth: How Do the Risks Compare?* New York: Maternity Center Association. (Full report available at www.maternitywise.org.)

13. Klaus, M., J. Kennell, and P. Klaus. (1998) *Your Amazing Newborn,* Reading, Ma: Perseus Books.

14. ———. (1998) *The Amazing Talents of the Newborn.* Johnson and Johnson Pediatric Institute.

15. American Academy of Pediatrics. (February 2005) "Policy Statement: Breastfeeding and the Use of Human Milk." *Pediatrics* 115, no. 2:496–506. (http://aappolicy.aappublications.org/cgi/content/full/pediatrics;115/2/496)

Chapter 12

1. Kitzinger, S. (2002) *Birth Your Way.* London: DK Publishers, 177.

2. Knoki-Wilson, U. (2003) "Keeping the Sacred in Childbirth Practices: Navajo Perspective." Lamaze International Annual Conference, Albuquerque, New Mexico.

3. Klaus, M. and J. Kennell. (1983) *Bonding: The Beginning of Parenting.* New American Library.

4. Gaskin, I. M. (2003) *Ina May's Guide to Childbirth.* New York: Bantam, 259.

5. Righard, L. and M. Alade. (1990) "Effect of delivery room routines on success of first breastfeed." *Lancet* 336, no. 8723:1105–107.

6. Matthiesen, A., et al. (2001) "Postpartum maternal oxytocin release by newborns: Effects of infant hand massage and suckling." *Birth* 28, no. 1:13–19.

7. Waldenstrom, U. and A. Swenson. (1991) "Rooming-in in the postpartum ward." *Midwifery* 7, no. 2:82–89; Keefe, M. (1987) "Comparison of neonatal nighttime sleep-wake patterns in nursery versus rooming-in environments." *Nursing Research* 36, no. 3:140–44; ——— (1988) "The impact of infant rooming-in on maternal sleep at night." *Journal of Obstetric, Gynecologic, and Neonatal Nursing* 17, no. 2:122–26.

8. Kushner, H. (2003) *The Lord Is My Shepherd: Healing Wisdom of the Twenty-Third Psalm.* New York: Knopf.

9. Crenshaw, J. (2003) *Care Practices that Promote Normal Birth: No Separation of Mother and Baby after Birth and Unlimited Opportunity for Breastfeeding.* Lamaze International: Lamaze Institute for Normal Birth.

10. Yamauchi, Y. and I. Yamanouchi. (1990) "The relationship between rooming-in/not rooming-in and breastfeeding variables." *Acta Pediatrica* 79, no. 11:1017–1022.
11. Syafruddin, M., et al. (1988) "A study comparing rooming-in with separate nursing." *Paediatrica Indonesiana* 79, no. 11:116–23.
12. Keefe, M. (1987) "Comparison of neonatal nighttime sleep-wake patterns in nursery versus rooming-in environments." *Nursing Research* 36, no. 3:140–44; ——— (1988) "The impact of infant rooming-in on maternal sleep at night." *Journal of Obstetric, Gynecologic, and Neonatal Nursing* 17, no. 2:122–26.
13. Prodomidis, M., et al. (1995) "Mothers touching newborns: A comparison of rooming-in versus minimal contact." *Birth* 22, no. 4:196–200; Klaus, M., et al. (1972) "Maternal attachment: Importance of the first postpartum days." *The New England Journal of Medicine* 286, no. 9:460–63; Norr, K., et al. (1989) "Early postpartum rooming-in and maternal attachment behaviors in a group of medically indigent primiparas." *Journal of Nurse Midwifery* 34, no. 2:85–91.
14. Enkin, M., et al. (2000) *A Guide to Effective Care in Pregnancy and Childbirth.* New York: Oxford University Press, chapter 33.
15. American Academy of Pediatrics. (1999). "Cord blood banking." *Pediatrics* 104, no. 1:116–18.
16. Dick-Reed, G. (2004 edition) *Childbirth without Fear: The Principles and Practice of Natural Childbirth.*
17. Enkin, M., et al. (2000) *A Guide to Effective Care in Pregnancy and Childbirth.* New York: Oxford University Press, chapters 44 and 46.
18. Gray, L., et al. (2002). "Breastfeeding is analgesic in healthy newborns." *Pediatrics* 4:590–95.
19. Academy of Breastfeeding Medicine. (1999) "Guidelines for Glucose Monitoring and Treatment of Hypoglycemia in Term Infants." (Available at www.bfmed.org/protocol/protocol.html.)
20. American Academy of Pediatrics. (1999) "Circumcision Policy Statement." (Available at www.aap.org.)
21. Ibid.
22. Gartner, M. and M. Herschel. (2000) "Jaundice and breastfeeding." *Pediatric Clinics of North America* 48, no. 2:389–97.
23. Klaus, M., J. Kennell, and P. Klaus. (2001) *Your Amazing Newborn.* Cambridge, Ma: Perseus, 52.
24. Ibid., 32–41.
25. Ibid., chapter 5.
26. Ibid., chapter 6.
27. Ibid., chapter 3.
28. Bell, S. and M. Ainsworth. (1973) "Infant crying and maternal responsiveness." *Child Development* 43:1171.
29. See note 23 above, 31.

Chapter 13

1. McKenna, J. "Cultural Influences on Infant Sleep." (www.attachmentparenting.org/cosleepmckenna.shtml)
2. McKenna, J., et al. (1997) "Bedsharing promotes breastfeeding." *Pediatrics* 100:214–19; McKenna, J. (1991) "Sleep and arousal patterns among co-sleeping mother-infant pairs: Implications for SIDS." *American Journal of Physical Anthropology* 83:331–37.
3. Academy of Breastfeeding Medicine. (2003) "Guidelines for Co-Sleeping and Breastfeeding." (www.bfmed.org/protocol/proto6.html)
4. McKenna, J. and S. Mosko. (1994) "Sleep and arousal, synchrony and independence: Nursing infants and mothers sleeping apart and together." *Acta Paediatrica* 397:94–102.
5. McKenna, J. (1991) "Sleep and arousal patterns among co-sleeping mother-infant pairs: Implications for SIDS." *American Journal of Physical Anthropology* 83:331–37.
   Fox, M. "Stressed Babies May Be Prone to Trouble Later." www.atlc.org (Alliance for Transforming the Lives of Children.)
7. Coburn, Jennifer, "The benefits of co-sleeping: Lower your baby's risk of stress disorders, SIDS and more," *The Compleat Mother* (www.breast-feeding.com)
8. Consumer Product Safety Commission. (October 1999) "Hazards for Babies on Adult Beds." Position paper in *The Archives of Pediatrics and Consumer Medicine.*
9. Sears, William, "Safe Co-Sleeping." (iparenting.com)
10. Newman, J. and T. Pitman. (2000) *The Ultimate Breastfeeding Book of Answers.* New York: Prena Publications.
11. American Academy of Pediatrics. (February 2005) "Policy Statement: Breastfeeding and the Use of Human Milk." *Pediatrics* 115, no. 2:496–506. (http://aappolicy.aappublications.org/cgi/content/full/pediatrics;115/2/496)
12. Ibid.
13. http://www.who.int/child-adolescent-health/NUTRITION/infant_exclusive.htm
14. Beck, K. (March/April 2004) "Baby fat: The new mom's struggle with body image" *Mothering* 123.
15. Rogers, F. (2003) *The World According to Mister Rogers: Important Things to Remember.* New York: Hyperion, 168.

RECOMMENDED RESOURCES

Books

Declercq, E., Sakala, C., Corry, M., et al. (2002) *Listening to Mothers: Report of the First U.S. Survey of Women's Childbirth Experiences*. New York: Maternity Center Association. (available at www.maternitywise.org)

DeVries, R. (2005) *A Pleasing Birth*. Philadelphia: Temple University Press.

England, P. and Horowitz, R. (1998) *Birthing from Within: An Extra-Ordinary Guide for Childbirth Preparation*. Partera Press.

Enkin, M., Keirse, M., Neilson, J. et al (2000) *A Guide to Effective Care in Pregnancy and Childbirth*. New York: Oxford University Press. (Full text of this book is available at www.maternitywise.org, or visit the Cochrane Library at www.cochrane.org.)

Gaskin, Ina May. (2003) *Ina May's Guide to Childbirth*. New York: Bantam Books.

Goer, H. and Wheeler, R. (1999) *The Thinking Woman's Guide to a Better Birth*. Perigee Books.

Kitzinger, S. (2002) *Birth Your Way*. DK Publishing.

Kitzinger, S. (2003). *The Complete Book of Pregnancy and Childbirth*. New York: Knopf.

Kitzinger, S. (2000) *Rediscovering Birth*. New York: Pocket Books

Klaus, M., Kennell, J., Klaus, P. (1998) *Your Amazing Newborn*. Perseus Books.

Klaus, M., Kennell, J., Klaus, P. (2002) *The Doula Book*. Cambridge, Ma.: Perseus Books.

La Leche League. (2004) *The Womanly Art of Breastfeeding*. Seventh Edition. La Leche League Publishing.

Lamaze International. (2003) *Promoting, Protecting and Supporting Normal Birth. Care Practice Position Papers*. (available at www.normalbirth.lamaze.org)

Maternity Center Association. (2004) *What Every Pregnant Woman Needs to Know About Cesarean Section*. (available at www.maternitywise.org and www.normalbirth.lamaze.org)

Newman, J. and Pitman, T. (2000) *The Ultimate Breastfeeding Book of Answers*. New York: Prima Publishing.

O'Mara, P. (2003) *Mothering Magazine's Having a Baby Naturally*. Atria Books.

Rooks, J. (1997) *Midwifery and Childbirth in America*. Philadelphia: Temple University Press.

Simkin, P., Whalley, J., and Keppler, A. (2001) *Pregnancy, Childbirth, and the Newborn*. Minnetonka, Mn.: Meadowbrook Press.

Tamaro, J. (1998) *So That's What They're For: Breastfeeding Basics*. Adams Media Corporation.

Videos

Many of these videos are used in Lamaze classes. Ask your childbirth educator about them.

Amazing Talents of the Newborn. (1998) with Marshall Klaus. Johnson and Johnson Pediatric Institute. Available at 877-JNJ-LINK, fax 877-565-3299, or www.jjpi.com. This video is less than $15 and well worth purchasing.

Celebrate Birth. Injoy Videos with Lamaze International. 800-326-2082. www.lamaze.org

Everyday Miracles. (a seven minute segment of *Celebrate Birth*) Injoy Videos with Lamaze International. 800-326-2082. You can view this video in its entirety on the Lamaze International website. www.lamaze.org

Open Minds to Birth. (2002) Vida Health Communications. www.vidahealth.com

Timeless Way: A History of Birth from Ancient to Modern Times. Injoy Videos. 800-326-2082

Gentle Birth Choices (1996) 800-641-baby

Follow Me Mum: The Key to Successful Breastfeeding. (2003) reblact@iinet.net.au. Available in the U.S. at the Lamaze Media Center.

The Real Deal on Breastfeeding. Available from www.realdealvideos.com

Infant Feeding Cues. (1998) www.mark-it-television.com

Comfort Measures for Childbirth. Penny Simkin. Injoy Videos. 800-326-2082.

Birth Day with Naoli Lopez and family. 1999 Sage Femme productions. Available at www.home-birthvideos.com or at the Lamaze International website, www.lamaze.org.

Organizations

American Academy of Pediatrics (AAP)
141 Northwest Point Boulevard
Elk Grove Village, IL 60007-1098
Phone: 847-434-4000
Fax: 847-434-8000
http://www.aap.org

American College of Nurse-Midwives (ACNM)
8403 Colesville Road, Suite 1550
Silver Spring, MD 20910-6374
Phone: 240-485-1800
Fax: 240-485-1818
http://www.midwife.org

Canadian Association of Midwives
http://www.canadianmidwives.org

Canadian Doula Association
4 Lamplight Bay
Spruce Grove, Alberta T7X 4N2
Phone: 780-962-1846
http://www.canadiandoulas.com

Canadian Paediatric Society
2305 St. Laurent Boulevard
Ottawa, Ontario K1G 4J8
Phone: 613-526-9397
Fax: 613-526-3332
http://www.cps.ca

Citizens for Midwifery
P.O. Box 82227
Athens, GA 30608
http://www.cfmidwifery.org

The Coalition for Improving Maternity Services (CIMS)
P.O. Box 2346
Ponte Vedra Beach, FL 32004
888-282-CIMS
Phone: 904-285-1613
Fax: 904-285-2120
http://www.motherfriendly.org

The Cochrane Library
http://www.cochrane.org

DONA International
P.O. Box 626
Jasper, IN 47547
Phone: 888-788-DONA
Fax: 812-634-1491
http://www.dona.org

International Cesarean Awareness Network (ICAN)
1304 Kingsdale Avenue
Redondo Beach, CA 90278
Phone: 800-686-ICAN or 310-542-6400
Fax: 310-542-5368
http://www.ican-online.org

International Lactation Consultant Association (ILCA)
1500 Sunday Drive, Suite 102
Raleigh, NC 27607
Phone: 919-861-5577
Fax: 919-787-4916
http://www.ilca.org

La Leche League International (LLLI)
P.O. Box 4079
Schaumburg, IL 60168-4079
Phone: 847-519-7730
Fax: 847-519-0035
http://www.lalecheleague.org

Lamaze International
2025 M Street NW, Suite 300
Washington, DC 20036
800-368-4404
http://www.lamaze.org

Maternity Center Association (MCA)
281 Park Avenue South, 5th Floor
New York, NY 10010
Phone: 212-777-5000
Fax: 212-777-9320
http://www.maternitywise.org

Midwives Alliance of North America (MANA)
4805 Lawrenceville Highway, Suite 116-279
Lilburn, GA 30047
Phone: 888-923-MANA (6262)
Fax: 417-777-6181
http://www.mana.org

Vaginal Birth After Cesarean (VBAC)
Nicette Jukelevics, MA, ICCE
Center For Family
24050 Madison Street, Suite 200
Torrance, CA 90505
310-375-3141
http://www.vbac.com

INDEX

A

B

C

Federal Drug Administration (FDA), 75
Female obstetricians, 49
Fertility, breastfeeding and, 217
Fetoscope, 116, 117
Fiji, 22
Finland, 15
Fluid intake
    during breastfeeding, 212
    during birth, 115–16
    during pregnancy, 36–37
FMLA. *See* Family and Medical Leave Act
    (FMLA) (1993)

G

Gaskin, Ina May, 11, 14, 35, 49, 124, 180, 227
Gender, knowing baby's, 76
Gentle Birth Choices (video), 142
Gestate, 27
Gestational diabetes, 78
Glucose screening, 190
Glucose tolerance test, 78
Guided imagery, 132–33
*A Guide to Effective Care in Pregnancy and
    Childbirth,* 15, 16, 21, 49, 56, 78

H

Haire, Doris, 14
Hall, Kathryn, 23, 83
Hearing, in newborn, 196
Heat/cold, pain perception and, 131
Hepatitis B vaccination, 190
Hinds, Josh, 220
Hodnett, Ellen, 229
Hofmeyr, G. Justus, 229
Home birth(s)
    advantages of, 58
    international support for, 14–15
    is as safe or safer than hospital births, 43–44
    making an informed decision on, 58–59
    midwive-attended births and, 47

personal account of, 60
    shift to hospital births from, 9–12
Hormonal shifts, 28
Hospital birth(s). *See also* Medical birth(s);
    Medical intervention(s)
    characteristics of, 53–54, 56
    having a comfortable environment for, 127
    lack of emotional and physical support for, 112
    mother-baby separation and, 182
    myths on, 43–44
    pain relief for, 45
    personal account of experience of, 55
    shift from home births to, 9–12
    time with your newborn after giving birth
        and, 178, 179
Hospitals
    childbirth classes at, 95
    doula programs in, 280
    midwife practices dictated by, 174–75
Husband-Coached Childbirth (Bradley), 13

I

Iatrogenic obstetric problems, 43–44
Iceland, 15
Immaculate Deception (Arms), 14
Induced labor, 106–8
    avoiding unnecessary, 150–51, 174–75
    communication with caregiver about, 173–74
    Lamaze philosophy on, 262
    normal labor with, 151
    number of women using, 5
    what to know about, 150
    when to use, 150
Induction, 243. *See also* Induced labor
Internal EFM, 116
International Cesarean Awareness Network
    (ICAN), 290
International Lactation Consultant Association
    (ILCA), 290
Intravenous (IV) fluids, 5, 116, 146–47

J

Japan, 15
Jaundice, 193–94

K

Karmel, Marjorie, 12
Kegel exercises, 153, 154
Keirse, Marc, 15, 229
Kennell, John, 114, 179, 279
Kitzinger, Sheila, 13, 59, 102, 106, 177
Klaus, Marshall, 179, 198, 279
Knoki-Wilson, Ursula, 179
Kroger, Mary, 108
Kushner, Harold, 183

L

Labor. *See also* Birth(s); Comfort measures, during
  labor; Contractions; Maternity care practices;
  Medical intervention(s)
  active, 98, 105
  comfort measures during.
    See Comfort measures, during labor
  early, 105–6
  impact of your surroundings on, 98
  learning from prior experience for, 156–59
  length of, 101
  listening to your body during, 88
  pain during. *See* Labor pain
  preparation for, 165–66. *See also* Birth plans
  pushing during. *See* Pushing
  self-trust and, 101–2
  unfolding differently than planned, 138–42
Labor contractions. *See* Contractions
Labor drugs, 16
  alternatives to, 44–45
  limiting, 134
  number of women using, 3

Labor pain. *See also* Comfort measures, during labor
  alternatives to drugs for, 3
  asking birth site about coping methods for, 53
  being realistic about, 135–36
Lamaze philosophy on, 259–60
  non-drug comfort methods for, 44–45
  purpose of, 100–101
  reducing perception of, 127–34
La Leche League, 162–63, 165, 169, 210, 222
La Leche League International (LLLI), 290
Lamaze Certified Childbirth Educator (LCCE), 93
Lamaze childbirth method
  in the 1960s, 91
  birth environment for, 262–63
  on emotional and physical support, 261
  has changed, vi, 259
  history of opposition to medical birth and, 12
  mother/baby connection and, 262
  philosophy of, 259, vii
  on relaxation and breathing, 260–61
  role of pain and, 259–60
Lamaze classes, 95
Lamaze Institute for Normal Birth, 21–22, 169
Lamaze International, 1, 12, 93, 290
Lamaze Parents (magazine), 163
Lamott, Anne, 215
Lanugo, 194
LCCE. *See* Lamaze Certified Childbirth
  Educator (LCCE)
Listening to Mothers survey (2002), 5, 21
  on birth outside a hospital, 56
  on epidural use, 119
  on freedom of movement during labor, 109
  on labor/birth interventions, 114–15
  on midwife-attended births, 47
Lovemaking, during pregnancy, 81

M

MANA. *See* Midwives Alliance of North
  America (MANA)
Massage, 133
Maternal/infant death rates
  medical technology's impact on, 18
  shift from home to hospital births and, 10, 11

N

O

P

Q

W

Y

Notes

Notes

Also from Meadowbrook Press

The Very Best Baby Name Book
This is the very best guide for helping you name your baby. It contains over 55,000 popular and unusual names from around the world, complete with origins, meanings, variations, and famous namesakes. It also includes the most recently available top 100 names for girls and boys, as well as over 250 helpful lists of names to consider and avoid.

First-Year Baby Care
This is one of the leading baby-care books to guide you through your baby's first year. It contains complete information on the basics of baby care, including bathing, diapering, medical facts, and feeding your baby. Newly revised.

Feed Me! I'm Yours
Parents love this easy-to-use, economical guide to making baby food at home. More than 200 recipes cover everything a parent needs to know about teething foods, nutritious snacks, and quick, pleasing lunches. Now recently revised.

Pregnancy Q & A
With quick, easy-to-understand answers to over 400 of the most frequently asked questions about pregnancy and childbirth, this book helps expectant mothers address the issues that medical providers don't always have time for. It also helps expectant parents communicate more effectively with their caregivers.

Getting Organized for Your New Baby
This interactive book is loaded with practical info and tips on conception, prenatal health, childbirth preparation, baby gear, household management, financial planning, childcare, celebrations, and life with baby. It's newly revised with the latest, greatest knowledge about pregnancy and parenting—plus key facts and resources to help busy parents-to-be make decisions.

The Simple Guide to Having a Baby
The authors of the best-selling *Pregnancy, Childbirth, and the Newborn* have written a simple, just-the-facts guide to pregnancy and childbirth for expectant parents who want only the most important, down-to-earth how-to information on pregnancy, childbirth, and newborn care.

Pregnancy, Childbirth, and the Newborn
More complete and up-to-date than any other pregnancy guide, this remarkable book is the "bible" for childbirth educators. It includes a thorough treatment of pregnancy tests, complications, infections, and medications and detailed advice on creating a birth plan.

**We offer many more titles written to delight, inform, and entertain.
To order books with a credit card or browse our full
selection of titles, visit our website at:**

www.meadowbrookpress.com
Meadowbrook Press • 5451 Smetana Drive • Minnetonka, MN • 55343 • 1-800-338-2232